The
MELT
Method

A Breakthrough Self-Treatment System
to Eliminate Chronic Pain, Erase the Signs of Aging,
and Feel Fantastic in Just 10 Minutes a Day!

Sue Hitzmann

with Debbie Karch

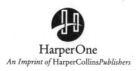

HarperOne
An Imprint of HarperCollinsPublishers

HarperOne

This book contains advice and information relating to health care. It is not intended to replace medical advice and should be used to supplement rather than replace regular care by your doctor. It is recommended that you seek your physician's advice before embarking on any medical program or treatment. All efforts have been made to ensure the accuracy of the information contained in this book as of the date of publication. The publisher and the author disclaim liability for any medical outcomes that may occur as a result of applying the methods suggested in this book.

Products, pictures, trademarks, and trademark names are used throughout this book to describe and inform the reader about various proprietary products that are owned by third parties. No endorsement of the information contained in this book is given by the owners of such products and trademarks, and no endorsement is implied by the inclusion of products, pictures, or trademarks in this book.

FIRST HARPERCOLLINS PAPERBACK EDITION PUBLISHED IN 2016

Designed by Terry McGrath
Photographs by Brian Leighton. Used by permission.
Illustrations by Gene Clark. Used by permission.

Library of Congress Cataloging-in-Publication Data

Hitzmann, Sue.
    The melt method : a breakthrough self-treatment system to eliminate chronic pain, erase the signs of aging, and feel fantastic in just 10 minutes a day! / by Sue Hitzmann.
        p. cm.
    ISBN 978–0–06–206536–0
    1. Chronic pain—Treatment—Popular works. 2. Stretching exercises—Popular works. 3. Self-care, Health—Popular works. I. Title.
RB127.H58 2012
616'.0472—dc23
                                        2012023457

    17 18 19 20 RRD (H) 10 9 8 7 6 5 4

Contents

Preface

I can't believe that I am writing the preface to the paperback edition of *The MELT Method.* So much has happened since the book first hit the stands January 2013.

Thanks to the support of an incredible community, the book has become a *New York Times* bestseller and been translated into nine languages. There are now over a thousand MELT instructors in fifteen countries worldwide, and hundreds of thousands of people have benefitted from MELT. To think, ten years ago it was just me in my office working with people one-on-one. Now I've had the opportunity to share MELT on *Dr. Oz, Rachael Ray, Good Morning America, Marilyn Denis, Nightline,* and *Home and Family,* publications such as the *New York Times* and *Los Angeles Times,* and countless other media. It has been such a thrill for me.

After appearing on the *Dr. Oz* show as the "woman who can MELT your pain away," I embarked on a yearlong thirty-city book tour that included over a hundred workshops across the U.S. and Canada. I got to teach people of all ages and fitness levels. There were men and women, from young athletes and injured yoga instructors to a ninety-four-year-old in a wheelchair whose granddaughter thought MELT might help the arthritis in her hands. There were people with severe diabetes, neuropathy, cancer, and debilitating back pain. Some limped in on walkers and crutches, others had prosthetic legs and missing fingers. I could hardly believe it when someone came with an oxygen tank rolling behind them and another with an IV attached to their arm. Some people drove more than three hours to take part in these workshops and many had suffered with chronic pain for years. In all, I MELTed thousands of people.

I shared my secrets to pain-free living at any age. I told them that there is a solution, a missing link within their body, and they would feel changes right then and there. And they did.

This book tour led to two important realizations: One was that anyone, in any condition, can benefit from MELT. No matter what age, health, or level of physical fitness, everyone who came in made positive changes. Even people who thought they had tried everything walked out feeling better than when they came in. MELT sparked hope and delivered help.

The second realization was that it was time to design a new roller specifically for the techniques of the MELT Method. So I set about developing the MELT Soft Roller. I reduced the circumference of the roller to 5 inches, an inch smaller than the one we had been using. It was perfect for MELT and completely unlike anything else on the market.

It's amazing how just a one-inch reduction in size allows so many more people to gain the benefits of MELT. Regardless of age, wellness, or height, the new roller accommodates people of all shapes and sizes without any additional props.

I also wanted a softer roller that would better mimic my light-touch, hands-on work. This is the first roller developed with memory foam and its unique density allows the connective tissue time to adapt while doing the sequences and makes better, faster changes than our old roller.

While I was at it, I also developed a soft half roller. The MELT Soft Half Roller is made of the same material but has a flat side to accommodate people who have trouble getting on the roller or who need more support. It has been such an asset to people with spinal diseases and disorders, Parkinson's and other neurological disorders, or who are pregnant. For more information about using MELT with these and other issues, see the newly revised Complementary Self-Treatment Plans in Chapter 14.

The MELT Method continues to grow and adapt, and this paperback edition reflects all the changes to the method. The smaller roller means that each move is done slightly differently to achieve the best results. This book includes all new images and revised instructions for each move.

In addition to the changes in the paperback, I'm tremendously excited to share scientific research that validates the MELT Method. On page 293, you can read about the study, which was called "Effect of the MELT Method on the Thoracolumbar Connective Tissue." It was conducted in partnership with the New Jersey Institute of Technology (NJIT) and led by a biomedical engineering grad student, Faria Sanjana, who was advised by Thomas Findley, Ph.D., and Hans Chaudhry, Ph.D. The study was presented at the 2015 Fascia Research Congress in Washington, DC, as well as the Fascia and Oncology Summit at Harvard University.

The objective of the study was to determine the effect of MELT on people with chronic low back pain and to study the changes MELT made in the connective tissue. The study found that MELT reduces chronic low back pain, increases flexibility, and initiates real change in the connective tissue, immediately and after four weeks. By contrast, the control group, which did not MELT, showed no improvement.

What's compelling is that these changes were made by the participants, on their own, with just the MELT tools, book, and DVD. What's even more powerful is that when you MELT you never do any of the techniques directly on the low back, yet significant changes in the low back tissue, pain, stiffness, and flexibility are achieved. This is the secret of MELT.

I am thrilled to have scientific evidence that supports the results I have seen every day for over a decade. MELT is a proven self-care tool for people with chronic pain so they can feel better without drugs or surgery.

You can try the Chronic Low Back Pain Self-Treatment Plan that was used in the study. It starts on page 272.

The MELT Method book has helped so many people get out of pain, and now it's your turn. I am delighted to share with you this new revised and comprehensive edition of *The MELT Method.* My journey continues and I'm excited to have you be a part of it.

Foreword

With the MELT Method, Sue Hitzmann introduces cutting-edge information and innovative techniques that anyone can use to get out of and stay out of pain. MELT also allows fitness and hands-on health professionals to give their clients tools to encourage proactive self-care. To my mind, this is the essence of Sue's contribution to the growing number of researchers currently studying human fascia, a long-neglected yet critically important aspect of human anatomy. For years she has been combining this important information with practical tools that anyone can use to take care of their own body in a new way. I admire any practice that helps people to help themselves. The MELT Method is just that.

Over the past decade I have watched Sue develop the MELT Method. Sue is relentless in her quest for knowledge, and is willing to refine her perspective over and over again when she gets new information. She is also tireless in her effort to understand complex scientific information, and then transform it into something simple and accessible. Sue pays attention to all the layers of the body, not just the ones that have already been written about. She teaches you how to take care of the body you actually have, as opposed to the "muscle body" upon which much of the fitness industry is focused. There is so much more to our bodies than just muscles, and Sue's efforts represent a great stride in expanding our awareness of our whole body.

The folks who join me to study anatomy in the laboratory are a very small, self-selected group. They are people who are willing to stretch themselves and their understanding well beyond their training. When Sue first joined me in the lab, she was already an established figure in the fitness world as well as an accomplished body-worker. She was a standout participant among the early adopters from the fitness industry. There are some people you meet, and you know on the spot that you will never forget them. Sue was such a person. Much to my delight, I have been privileged to know her ever since that first course she joined "way back when." What I remember of her from that first week we spent together in the lab was that she was on fire! Her bright eyes and intense curiosity demonstrated her complete engagement with the experience, and her palpable excitement for her discoveries. This lady had volumes of energy for her work, a vibrant personality, and a genuine enthusiasm for the process we were engaged in. She spoke to me as if she were on the brink of discovery. She was also clearly blessed with all the drive it takes to see a complex inquiry through to the end.

The first time I got to see Sue share the MELT message with a group was at a large fitness conference in New York City. While hearing Sue teach, my respect for her method grew. She systematically taught us how to self-assess our alignment, develop our body awareness, and increase our consciousness of the fascial system and how it related to what we were feeling. Then she offered simple, "do-able" techniques with little balls and soft rollers so that we could gently and effectively initiate changes for the better. She placed great emphasis on the gentleness required to effect positive change in our body, tossing aside decades of that insidious "no pain, no gain" mantra. This alone does us all a great service.

A couple of years ago I went out for a walk with my son, who was twelve at the time. We didn't get a hundred yards down the street when he complained about pain in his foot and ankle. We went back to the house and, thinking of Sue, I told my son that I was pretty sure I had a way to help him. I am trained in multiple hands-on healing modalities, and surely could have done my son some good with a manual therapy session. This time, though, I wanted him to know that he could take care of himself. I popped in Sue's Hand and Foot Treatment DVD, handed him the balls, and left him to it. I peeked in once or twice and saw him following Sue's straightforward instructions. Afterward, I asked him how it went, and he was happy to announce that the pain was gone. What thrilled me most was not that he was out of pain, but that he learned he could do that for himself.

Another thing I love about Sue's work is that she knows that the body is not a machine and that health requires more than merely fixing mechanical problems. Our bodies have ultra-sophisticated chemical, electrical, and energetic communication systems that need to be supported as well. When we open these channels of communication, we re-establish a baseline experience that feels good.

Sue's method always maintains a healthy respect for your body's own voice up front. She would rather have us whisper good feelings to the delicate, fluid tissues of the body than shout at them with even more pain signals. Based on my own decades-long study of the body, that is a program I can get behind. The intelligence of the body deserves our utmost consideration. Our bodies are not the enemy when we are in pain. Our bodies are on our side. Sue's program aligns with that fact and takes full advantage of the wisdom and subtle communication systems of the body for our own good.

The depth of Sue's MELT Method comes in large part from the fact that it is grounded in her own personal experience of self-healing. Sue is an enthusiastic explorer of her own body, to which she listens attentively. The importance of her work relies on careful attention to the needs of the body and its true structure, anatomy, and physiology. Translating cutting-edge science into a safe, practical, universally accessible application is no simple task, yet in the MELT Method, that's exactly what Sue has done.

—Gil Hedley, Ph.D., creator of Integral Anatomy

Introduction

For as long as I can remember, I've had the ability to feel the subtle vibrations that exist in all living things. When I touch a person, an animal, or a tree, if I focus my attention, I physically sense vibrations with my hands.

When I was a little girl, my father said this ability was weird and not to tell anyone because it would scare them. When I told my mom, she took me to the doctor's office. The doctor offered to cut some of the nerves in my hands to see if that would stop it from happening. Fortunately my mom thought that cutting into my hands to stop me from talking about it was a bit radical. She asked if it bothered me or got in the way of doing anything, and when I said no, she told me to ignore it and maybe it would go away.

My great-grandmother, however, told me that what might seem like a curse could become a blessing if I could learn what it was. She told me to keep it to myself until I found someone who could tell me how to use it. So I kept it to myself for many, many years.

When I was little, I was frequently grounded and sent to my room, where the only things I had to occupy me were fairy tales and the *Encyclopaedia Britannica.* I became fascinated with anatomy—I got the idea that it could give me the answer to what I felt in my hands.

I was always full of questions. I remember asking my father why there was so little in the encyclopedia about the nervous system. He answered, "How much do you need to know about the nervous system?" I didn't tell him that I thought I had found what I was feeling in my hands—nerve impulses.

Not long after, we were at the library. My dad pointed at the card catalog and said, "If you want to know more, use your brain and find a book that will teach you." (Can you imagine a time before the instant information of the Internet?)

When I was around twelve years old, my mother took me to Spa Lady, the gym she belonged to. The ladies there wore leotards and legwarmers. Seeing them dancing to loud music, smiling, and cheering each other on immediately enamored me.

My mom bought me *Jane Fonda's Workout Record,* and I soon became obsessed with the *20 Minute Workout* and every morning aerobics show on PBS. I aspired to be like the women I saw in movies like *Perfect* and *Flashdance.*

My first job was as an aerobics teacher at the local YMCA, when I was just sixteen. I became involved in every school sport possible. Once I was in college, I realized I could make money as a competitive cyclist, and I paid for most of my undergraduate tuition with my winnings.

I thought my life's path would be in film and theater, and I pursued a master's degree in film at New York University. When I lost my job as an assistant casting director, my dad sent me $200 and told me to go to the gym while looking for a new job because I was always happiest there. Not long after, I started teaching group exercise again, got certified as a personal trainer, and changed my master's study to exercise science. I have to admit I looked like a bodybuilder, and I certainly exercised like one. The other trainers at the gym called me Diesel. I was in deep.

I quickly became a well-known fitness professional with a reputation for making people suffer and sweat. At one point I was teaching twenty-eight classes—step and high-impact aerobics, body sculpting, boot camp, and indoor cycling—each week. I became a host for CRUNCH TV on ESPN and was known for being the "smartest girl in fitness with a body to prove it." I weighed 130 pounds, had 11 percent body fat, and was on the cover of *Muscle & Fitness Magazine.* I had one of the bestselling fitness videos of all times, *Crunch: Boot Camp Training,* and was a regular presenter at national fitness conventions. By all measures, I was in perfect health and a success. I had made it.

At the same time, I was taking every fitness and rehabilitation workshop and certification I had time for, in addition to my graduate coursework. I started asking more people if they felt these mysterious vibrations under the skin. I felt like the young bird in the children's book asking anyone and everyone, "Are you my mother?"

I took a risk and asked my teacher of neuromuscular therapy, Leon Chaitow, about the vibrations I could feel. He simply said, "There are many vibrations in the body."

Then one morning I woke up with a pain in my right heel. I iced, stretched, and rested as much as I could. I strengthened. I did everything I knew to do. Nothing helped! If anything, most of these things seemed to make it worse.

It got to the point where my foot hurt twenty-four hours a day. The pain was so intense that it woke me up at night and exhausted me during the day. I even remember having to crawl to the bathroom in the middle of the night.

I asked every mentor, teacher, and colleague I knew what I could do to resolve my pain. I found no real answers. In fact, almost everyone told me they were in pain too and had managed to live with it. Top New York City doctors didn't have any answers. I was in pain and afraid that if it didn't go away soon, my career would be at risk. I became very depressed.

After a friend's dog head-butted me in the face, leaving my upper lip completely numb, another friend recommended that I see a craniosacral therapist. In a single session, not only did the numbness in my lip go away, but the pain in my foot also literally vanished. I called the therapist the next day to find out what she had done.

In our conversation, I asked her if she felt vibrations when she touched people, and she actually knew what I was talking about. She said, "Yes. Can you? If you do, then you should learn how to use this skill."

So I did. I remember crying during my first craniosacral training. I was finally learning a method of accessing, influencing, and rebalancing a vibrational rhythm. For the first time in my life, I didn't feel strange because of what I could feel. That was it. I had found my calling in hands-on bodywork.

I opened a private practice in New York City, and I worked on anyone and everyone to build my skill of manipulating these vibrations to help restore balance in the body. For the next eight years, I studied, trained, and exchanged ideas with the creators of multiple modalities and read every relevant research paper available. I honed my skills, working on hundreds of people: adults, teens, children, and infants. Now, fifteen years later, I can confidently call myself an expert in hands-on bodywork. Sometimes I still surprise myself in what I can feel when I put my hands on people.

I researched and learned multiple light touch techniques. Although each modality focused on sensing and manipulating the rhythm and vibration of specific parts of the body, none of them identified the continuous whole body vibration I could sense ever since I was a little girl. As I continued to work on clients, I would begin my sessions just focusing on the whole body vibration I didn't have a name for. I had noticed that my clients who had pain and other chronic issues had a vibration that seemed slow and interrupted, whereas my clients without these issues had a vibration that had consistent, whole body movement. I wondered if I could use the same light touch I had learned to influence the movement of this vibration and create positive change. When I tried this, I found that supporting the movement of this vibration helped people feel better immediately and it improved many different issues, including—and most noticeably—a reduction or elimination of pain. My clients would return stating they had much less pain, and they noted many systemic changes. I knew I was on to something big. I made this discovery about four years into my manual therapy practice and I quickly became known for getting people out of pain, even when nothing else worked.

That same year, 2001, the World Trade Center towers were attacked. As I live in New York City, many of my friends, clients, and neighbors were directly affected by this event. It gave me an intense understanding of the effects of post-traumatic stress disorder. It also gave me an understanding of the effects of stress on the nervous system and the body-wide vibration that I was starting to understand.

One day, a colleague said, "Do you know Gil Hedley?" Without warning, my life was about to take another dramatic turn. Gil is a theologian and Rolfer who has become an anatomist. He developed his own human dissection method of removing tissues layer by layer, from the skin to the organs and bones. His intention is to examine the connections in the body rather than studying only the separate parts, as dissections are traditionally done.

I took his six-day dissection course, and on the first day, my entire knowledge of anatomy and the human form was completely turned inside out. While dissecting the individual layers of the body, I saw for the first time how all the parts connected. Gil introduced me to the connective tissue system, and suddenly the vibrations I was feeling had a physical, tangible explanation.

Once I saw the connective tissue system, I had to know more! This relatively unknown aspect of the human body intuitively made so much sense to me. It was the missing piece from my education in academia, fitness, and manual therapy, yet I had been working on it for years.

I searched through my library of academic and manual therapy texts and training manuals. I scoured the latest editions of standard medical references and scientific journals. I asked my mentors and teachers for any written materials or research, but I couldn't find anything beyond some limited views of connective tissue's relationship to muscle or the long-held belief that this tissue was nothing more than a nonliving packing material.

Gil pointed me to research online that could better explain the vibration I was sensing. I was ecstatic. Although the scientific language used in the text was way over my head, I had such a strong desire to learn that I persevered. I spent endless hours reading complex scientific studies and research papers. At my side at all times were at least two science books or journals, a dictionary, and the Internet so that I could translate the scientific jargon. After I understood one research paper, I would look at other authors referenced in the bibliography and review their research too. Ultimately I found the researchers who pioneered fascial science.

Looking back, I have to laugh at how bold and fearless I was. I called and wrote the researchers directly to ask questions and, to my surprise, they answered. I believe that the biggest reason they gave me the time of day was that I could speak their language and had enormous respect for their research. My ability to discuss the molecular components such as myofibroblasts, glycoaminoglycans, and mechanoreceptors as well as the theories of mechanotransduction and piezoelectricity seemed to catch their attention. After talking for a while, they would invariably ask, "Who are you? What is your background?"

My anatomy and physiology background helped me, yet most of what I was learning and discussing was beyond my schooling or anything I had learned professionally. It was so mentally stimulating to have the opportunity to talk with the pioneering researchers as they were finding ways to test their theories. I was at the right place at the right time to enter the backdoor of this sanctum. I'm still amazed that one of the top researchers, Robert Schleip, came to New York City from Germany for the purpose of experiencing MELT and to talk with me about his research.

My background is not in research. I hold no Ph.D. or medical license, yet my love of human science and how it works has influenced me to spend over two decades learning anything and everything about the human body. I never wanted to sit behind a microscope all day long or study algorithms or work tirelessly to develop research. Yet I can't help but read countless research papers, books, and journals and then proceed to call the researchers (who are delightful, kind, amazing people more than happy to direct me to more research and more researchers!).

My independent study of neurological and fascial science and the enthusiastic embrace of the research community validated and fueled my hands-on work and the development of MELT. The existence of research that was directly related to what I was pursuing bolstered my confidence and motivated me to keep going.

As I made new observations in my classes and with my clients, I kept talking to the researchers. Their work informed mine, and at times, mine even informed theirs. Participating in the emergence of this new field of human science has been the most intellectually and creatively stimulating opportunity of my life.

The word spread to the point where I could not see all the people who wanted appointments with me. When I started to develop at-home techniques for my clients, it not only had the unintended benefit of transitioning them out of my office quicker so I could see new clients, it also reduced the toll that my hands-on work took on me.

I decided that this technique needed a name, and I wanted a word that expressed what I was trying to achieve with the connective tissue. I thought *melt* was a perfect fit. In addition to evoking the feeling of relaxation, the definition of the word *melt* was ideal: to change a solid into a liquid and blend or merge. Many techniques in fitness have acronyms, so I thought I needed one too. I brainstormed a lot of different combinations and decided that M.E.L.T. would stand for Myofascial Energetic Length Technique. As MELT has evolved, the method has outgrown the acronym. For one thing, it's now clear that it affects the entire connective tissue system, not just the fascia around and inside muscles. Still today when people try it for the first time, they say the name seems perfect.

Although I am no longer ripped with muscle and do not lift nearly the weight I once did, I still love to work out, teach indoor cycling, run, and lift weights. Thanks to MELT, I didn't have to give up anything I loved to have a pain-free body—and neither do you.

When I started teaching MELT in fitness clubs, it was so exciting to be able to create the same types of changes in a room full of people that I did one person at a time in my office. And they could do it to themselves.

Since then, I have trained over a thousand MELT instructors and practitioners and together we have helped tens of thousands with MELT's Hands-Off Bodywork. I never set out to create a method. The organic unfolding that led to the creation of MELT can be traced back to the vibrations I felt with my hands when I was a little girl.

My great-grandmother was right. My curse has become my greatest blessing, and I am grateful and honored to share it with you.

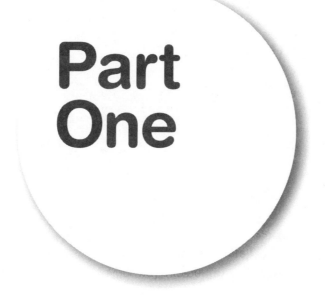

Part
One

1

What *Really* Causes Pain?

Imagine this is your average day: you wake up in the morning after a great night's sleep. You feel refreshed, alert, and ready for your day. You walk with a bounce in your step, and your body feels light and vibrant. You smile. People mention how great you look and notice your boundless energy. The demands of your day don't overwhelm you, and stress rolls off your shoulders. It's effortless to connect with and be generous to your loved ones—and even to strangers. You sit, stand, and move in a relaxed way. You are not nagged by thoughts about how your body feels. You live in the present moment and easily say yes to new experiences.

Is this what your average day feels like? If you have pain, your answer is probably no. Maybe you don't call it pain. Maybe you call it discomfort, tension, or something that doesn't feel quite right. Being pain-free is a necessary component of good health. It's much easier to live a good life when you feel good. You may attribute how you feel to your lifestyle, age, or genetics. But now it's time to look at the whole picture.

I am here to tell you that you can live pain-free.

I don't want you to have to waste another day or dollar on trying to figure out why you have pain or discomfort. I'm going to teach you how to sense it, address it, and eliminate it. The solution is simple. I am going to share a new way of looking at the body's design and teach you how to use that information so you never have to look for another pain solution again. Even if you feel you have the right diet, water, supplements, exercise routine, meditation practice, mattress, massage therapist, and integrative or holistic doctors—you haven't tried this yet. I've got the secret to pain-free living, and it's within you.

For all of the billions of dollars spent on trying to eliminate pain and discomfort, you would think that the mystery of pain would have been solved by now. But the statistics show otherwise. The National Institutes of Health (NIH) reports that pain affects more Americans than diabetes, heart disease, and cancer do combined. It is the most common reason individuals seek medical care, costing Americans more than $100 billion each year. According to the American Pain Society, pain is the second leading cause of medically related work absenteeism, resulting in more than 50 million lost workdays each year. The NIH also reports that one in three Americans suffers from some type of chronic or lasting pain, and approximately two-thirds have been living with this pain for more than five years. That means that more than 100 million people in the United States are living with chronic pain—and, based on my practice and experience, I believe that this estimate is low.

Pain affects your quality of life on every level. One in three Americans loses more than twenty hours of sleep each month because of pain, according to the National Sleep Foundation. It's not surprising that pain and discomfort can cause anxiety, worry, and mood swings. Ask your coworkers, friends, or family whether they have chronic pain. You'll probably be amazed by the number of people you know who spend a lot of time and energy worrying about, managing, or trying to ignore pain. I've found that many people who make investments of time, energy, and money to do all the "right," healthy things still experience daily pain and discomfort.

▶ You Can Live Without Pain

Living a pain-free life is an amazing feeling. Ironically, it is hard to truly appreciate how great it feels to be pain-free unless you've experienced an ongoing ache, pain, or discomfort. I know about enduring pain firsthand. Over a decade ago, I was at the height of success in my career as an international fitness presenter and instructor and seemed to be in perfect health. Yet I had debilitating pain in my right foot. I had a master's degree in exercise science, multiple fitness certifications, advanced training in neuromuscular therapy, and experience as a research intern in kinesiology at New York–Presbyterian/Weill Cornell Medical Center. I thought I knew everything there was to know about the human body and about how to stay fit, healthy, and active. Yet I couldn't get relief or answers from anyone, including New York City doctors.

I was only in my twenties. My fitness career was threatened, and my quality of life was in decline. I continually asked myself, my peers, and my teachers, "Why is this happening? What is causing all this pain? Is my body failing me?" My search for understanding and my quest to heal my own pain led me to an unexpected answer: My body wasn't failing me; it was desperately trying to get my attention. I did not recognize what I now know to be easily recognizable signs. I knew so much about the human body, yet the solution to my pain had nothing to do with what I knew.

Ultimately, I found therapies that helped heal my pain, yet the methods were unexplainable scientifically. I needed to understand what was creating the positive changes in my body, so the search for the true cause of pain continued. I stumbled upon research that was just starting to answer my questions. It was a revelation to me. My questions had answers, and the answers were based on new science. It was as if I had cracked an egg I had been tapping for years. The discoveries and insights that led to the resolution of my pain also changed my career and led me to a new, overriding question:

How do I live a healthy, active, pain-free lifestyle for my whole life?

Sharing the answers to this question has become my purpose in life. When I resolved my own pain, I felt a calling to help others do the same. I shifted my focus from training people to be fit to helping people feel better. I became a manual thera-pist, which means that I use hands-on, physical interventions. In my private practice, I've treated pain associated with practically every disease, disorder, and chronic condition that has a name—as well as some that don't. I can't even count the number of people I've seen who are dealing with a less-than-full recovery from acute circum-stances such as injury, childbirth, or surgery.

Regardless of their age, body type, activity level, financial means, stress level, occupation, condition, or symptoms, all my clients had pain. What was surprising to me was that the simple solution I had discovered for pain also had a positive effect on their overall health. Regardless of their history, their bodies started to find their own path to healing. Instead of having to stop doing the activities they enjoyed, my clients could return to doing the things they loved. This is one of the most rewarding aspects of my work—helping people get their lives back.

▶ The *Real* Secret

The secret to living the pain-free life you deserve is to directly address the real cause of your pain. I believe that the actual reason your physical pain started is a much more important factor than what symptoms you're feeling or how long your pain has lasted. Understanding the true reason for your pain will profoundly affect your ability to resolve your symptoms and live pain-free. This information—and a specialized soft body roller, small balls, and a little time—is your pathway to pain-free living.

❱ The Big Ouch

Looking back, it's easy for me to remember the events that caused me acute pain. When I burned my hand while making angel food cake with my grandmother, I experienced acute pain for the first, but not the last, time. There was the time I bashed my finger with a hammer, when I smashed my nose into a sliding glass door, and when I broke my ankle falling out of a tree. When I was eighteen, I ran my truck into a tree when I swerved to avoid hitting a deer. I totaled the truck and had quite a head injury to prove it. I've broken numerous fingers and toes and have had more sports injuries than I can count. Most recently, I broke my toe when I accidentally kicked the leg of a coffee table. I'm sure you've experienced moments such as these, ones you wish you could take back because afterward you experienced acute pain.

The cause of acute pain is very simple. It involves a one-time event or trauma that produces an acute injury with accompanying intense, sometimes excruciating, take-your-breath-away pain. Your nervous system uses this pain to get your attention in order to avoid further injury. However, just because pain comes on suddenly doesn't mean it's acute pain. You can have excruciating pain without an actual traumatic event.

When you have an acute injury, you should immediately call your doctor or go to the emergency room. Following an acute injury, pain usually decreases and becomes a more subtle message that you need to protect and rest the injured area. Ideally the injury heals, your body recovers, and the pain signal is no longer needed. However, when pain from an acute trauma isn't fully resolved by the body's own healing process, it becomes a chronic pain.

❱ "Normal" Discomfort

The discomfort that seems to be the most pervasive yet mystifying for people is chronic pain. Before the pain becomes chronic, it usually starts as what most people would describe as a "normal," everyday discomfort. You've probably experienced feelings of stiffness, soreness, throbbing, heaviness, tenderness, and tightness on occasion. When these sensations become a daily discomfort over a prolonged period of time, you realize the pain isn't going away. You now have chronic pain.

Although my first chronic pain was in my foot, I had experienced many discomforts. I was no stranger to stiffness in my knee, tightness in my shoulders, cramping in my hands, and aching in my low back. I assumed these day-to-day nuisances were all part of "being fit." I had bought into the "no pain, no gain" message, believing that if I didn't have some discomfort, I wasn't working hard enough. I look back now and see just how much wasted effort I put into trying to ignore or manage my pain.

What I thought were normal discomforts, I now identify as pre-pain symptoms. Have you had any pre-pain symptoms lately?

- When you woke up today, did your body feel stiff?

- Do you feel achy when you get out of a chair or after exercise?

- Does walking up a flight of stairs make you wish for an elevator?

- Do you find yourself adjusting, stretching, cracking, or rubbing your neck or back to try to relieve tension?

- Do you experience stiffness or swelling in your hands and feet?

- Do you have unexplainable aches or stiffness in multiple areas of your body?

These are just a few common pre-pain symptoms. What I've seen in every single one of my clients who has chronic pain is that they also experience one or more other symptoms. See if you've ever experienced any of these for more than a week at a time.

- Do you have difficulty falling asleep or staying asleep?

- Do you have gas or indigestion, no matter what you eat?

- Do you feel exhausted or have a mild headache in the afternoon?

- Do you find yourself exhausted by midday?

- Do you wake up with anxiety or have mood swings?

- Do you feel bloated or struggle with your weight?

Many people consider these symptoms to be normal. Yet, what happens when mild symptoms occur regularly for weeks or months, or one pre-pain symptom turns into three? Then what?

If you feel stiff and achy, have trouble sleeping, or feel bloated *over weeks or months,* or if you have more than one of these pre-pain symptoms, you might have an illness or disease. So it's important to visit your doctor to have your symptoms evaluated and rule out whether or not these lingering symptoms are being caused by an underlying illness or disease. If illness and disease are ruled out, the standard medical treatment for lingering symptoms is usually medication and the underlying cause is not identified or addressed. With only this approach, chronic pain is almost always inevitable, and pain medication or pain "management" solutions to decrease the symptom of pain are the only medical option.

I have a better solution that treats the underlying cause of pre-pain symptoms. In my practice, I have seen many clients who have multiple symptoms that are seemingly unrelated. Yet, in treating the underlying cause with MELT, I've helped them eliminate chronic pain and all their pre-pain symptoms.

The important point is: pain and discomfort are your body's way of trying to get your attention so you will take care of something. I'm going to help you discover what your "something" is and show you how easy it is to take care of it. In other words, I'll help you finally be free of your pain and discomfort! Whether your level of pain is interfering with your life or you only have occasional aches or stiffness, I am here to tell you that you don't have to accept pain as a normal part of aging or active living. MELT will help you resolve these pre-pain symptoms so you can live without chronic pain.

▶ Acute Misunderstanding

Most people believe that *any pain* that starts with an intense, recognizable event is acute pain. However, in my practice, I have heard countless stories of sudden, intense pain not caused by an acute injury. In every story, the people could recall when the pain started and what they were doing at the time. Yet the activity in no way matched the intensity of the sudden pain. There you are: you tie your shoe, reach into your trunk for groceries, get out of bed, do an exercise or yoga pose you've done a hundred times before, climb the stairs, step out of the bathtub, stand up from your desk chair, or bend over to pick up a pencil, and all of a sudden you feel a pain that makes you freeze in your tracks. This is when my clients call me and say, "Sue, help! I don't know what I did, but I can barely move my head/neck/arm/back/knee/foot. I am in so much pain. I don't know what to do!"

Although the pain came on suddenly, I don't think these examples fall under the category of acute pain. In my view, this is a type of chronic pain that has been lurking, slowly building in the background, waiting to reveal itself. This is what I call sudden chronic pain, and it is far more common than acute pain. The reason it's critical to make the distinction between sudden chronic and acute pain is that sudden chronic pain will almost always become a full-blown chronic pain that will either come and go or come and stay. What's tricky is that acute pain and sudden chronic pain can have the same level of intensity. Yet picking up a pencil, climbing stairs, and getting out of bed are not acute traumatic events. These everyday events are merely the tipping point for your overstressed body. So what is causing this sudden chronic pain?

▶ The Real Cause

Whether a chronic ache or pain comes on suddenly or slowly, the source is the same—repetition. Don't get me wrong. Repetition—or the idea of practice, practice, practice—can be a very good thing. Repetition is what has made me the best teacher and bodyworker I can be. As I continue to repeat these activities, I can improve my skills and be even better. Repetition is a normal, useful part of life, not something you could or should try to eliminate. That said, the primary cause of chronic and sudden chronic pain is repetitive movements and postures, not aging or muscle tension, as many people believe. But you don't have to figure out how to eliminate your repetitive habits: by adding MELT, you can help undo repetition's negative effects.

Think about it: what repetitive movements (such as typing or jogging) and repetitive postures (such as sitting or standing) do you do regularly in your day or week? How many hours a day do you sit? The time spent sitting when you eat, drive your car, work at your desk, watch TV, and read in bed really adds up. If sitting isn't your repetition, what is? Is it standing at work all day? Carrying around your kids or chasing after them? Remember, I'm not asking you to give up anything in your life to get out of pain. I'm going to ask you to add ten minutes, three times a week.

The component in your body that supports you and keeps you stable is your connective tissue, scientifically known as fascia. The connective tissue surrounds and supports all aspects of your body, including your muscles, bones, nerves, and organs. It's a three-dimensional web that seamlessly connects everything from head to toe and skin to bones. There is more connective tissue in your body than anything else—it is everywhere. The connective tissue creates a flexible framework that compartmentalizes, separates, and connects everything in your body. Collectively, the connective tissue is in fact a system that provides a seamless continuum throughout your body.

What is far more mind-blowing is that research is finding evidence that the connective tissue system is intelligent and adaptable. We have only just begun to understand and define the many functions that this powerful system serves in the body.

In my traditional schooling, I learned what everyone does: that connective tissue is a passive packing material in the body. The connective tissue has long been viewed as having the singular job of just passively protecting the important structures it surrounds, like Styrofoam peanuts do. But the connective tissue system—not your muscles and bones, as many people think—provides the body its architectural stability. This tissue is constantly morphing and adapting to your movements and positions to support your joints, bones, and organs. The connective tissue can only do its job when it has an adequate amount of fluid.

The repetition of daily living causes connective tissue to become dehydrated from excessive compression, pull, and friction. Dehydration makes connective tissue less supportive, responsive, and adaptable, which causes strain in muscles, compression in joints, and a disconnect in the communication required for any bodily movement or position, repetitive or not. This isn't just about drinking water, it's about getting the fluid moving in the tissues. Connective tissue dehydration is the underlying cause of strain and pain in the body as well as the catalyst for your pre-pain symptoms.

This may seem odd, but to the body, activity and inactivity are both dehydrating. If you're sitting at a desk for hours at a time, your own body weight is compressing and dehydrating your butt and thighs while your posture is pulling on and dehydrating the tissue from your head to your tailbone. If you're training for a marathon, the repetitive motion of running compresses and causes friction in your joints and pulls on tendons, ligaments, and lines of connective tissue. What creates this dehydration may be different, but in both cases, connective tissue loses its vital fluid. The fact of the matter is: life is dehydrating.

This is not the bad news. It's the good news. The remarkable new information that I have to share with you about connective tissue is that the tissue itself is *treatable* and *easily accessible.* New research has shown that this tissue is not passive as once believed; it plays an active, vital role in our health and overall well-being. The missing link to living pain-free is to erase the negative effects of repetition by treating your connective tissue. I'm going to teach you how easy it is to restore the fluid state of your connective tissue with MELT. It's this tissue that needs your attention whether you currently experience pain or pre-pain symptoms or you have no body issues and feel great.

Regardless of whether you have chronic, sudden chronic, or acute pain, the way out of pain is the same—and it's surprisingly simple. I'm going to teach you how you can keep your connective tissue hydrated and healthy in just ten minutes a day. Whether you want to resolve the pain you have or keep pain out of your life, you will now be able to access the underlying cause. The first time you try MELT, you will feel a difference. The control is now in your hands. Once you are living with more ease, you'll wish you had known about the restorative capability of connective tissue a long time ago. I know I did.

▶ Connective Tissue and Your Nervous System

You probably don't realize how much your whole body gets involved in every movement you make. The amount of preparation, communication, and micro-adjustments that occur before, during, and after every movement you make is almost greater than we can comprehend. The connective tissue system plays an essential role in your ability to move or remain still. Every minute of every day, your connective tissue is helping your body to do what you ask of it while also protecting your joints, bones, and organs.

Unlike muscle, connective tissue doesn't receive input from the brain or nervous system in order to adapt to your movement. The connective tissue independently plays its active role in stabilizing your joints and supporting and protecting all parts of your body so movement doesn't cause damage. This independent ability is part of why we haven't understood the connective tissue's capabilities and purpose. However, the connective tissue system does not do this alone. This system is inherently linked to a specific component of the nervous system—the autonomic nervous system—and together they regulate posture, joint position, and mind-body communication. The interdependent relationship between the connective tissue system and the autonomic nervous system, or what I call the neurofascial system, is what allows proper muscle contraction to occur.

Your nervous system relies on the fluid state of the connective tissue system for proper communication. The part of the nervous system that relies on the healthy, fluid state of your connective tissue the most is your sensory nerves. This is because the majority of your sensory nerve endings are found in the connective tissue system. If the connective tissue system is dehydrated, it can alter sensory nerve transmission. These nerves play a vital role in creating accurate, seamless movement. The sensory nerves also transmit pain signals, including when your connective tissue is unable to adequately support your joints, nerves, muscles, and bones because of dehydration.

These discoveries about the connective tissue system and the nervous system streamline the understanding of the cause and treatment of pain. When you have pain, you need to treat the connective tissue *system* as a whole. What has made the topic of pain seem so complicated is all the money, time, and effort spent on pain "solutions" that don't solve the problem. Looking to medicine, rehabilitation, exercise, and ineffective gimmicks and gadgets for the solution has been ineffective for so many people. The fact that chronic pain is so prevalent means something is missing from how we care for our bodies. Even the best exercise and nutritional habits can't restore the fluid state of the connective tissue system or rebalance your nervous system. But MELT can and does.

This new information about the human body turned my world upside down. My education, profession, and belief system were challenged. I had to learn the hard way that exercise, conventional medicine, and rehabilitation focused on treating the symptoms instead of the cause. Furthermore, utilizing these conventional approaches allows the connective tissue to stay dehydrated and pain to become chronic. I had to shift my thinking about anatomy, exercise, medicine, pain, and health to learn and benefit from the untapped potential of connective tissue. I want to provide you with the benefit of my journey of discovery.

▶ Reality Check: Medical Treatment of Pain

Because I've seen so many clients with pain caused by a variety of issues from migraines to cancer, I've had a firsthand look at the wonders of modern medicine.

Whether you've had a life-threatening injury or illness, or you've had a cut or minor infection, doctors can offer proven cures. Unfortunately, chronic pain is in a category outside of this curable realm. Yet pain of any kind is the number-one reason people consult a physician. When there's no immediate reason for pain, as there would be with acute trauma or injury, a doctor will look to rule out illness or disease as the underlying cause. When you break your wrist or are diagnosed with a tumor, there are definitive options for medical treatment.

Disease and acute trauma are at opposite ends of the medical spectrum. In between these two ends of the spectrum is a huge gap of chronic issues, ailments, and symptoms, including chronic pain. The treatment protocol for unexplainable pain symptoms that are in the "chronic gap" is frequently a guessing game of pharmaceutical trial and error or exploratory surgical procedures. There is also a huge gap between the options of pain medication or surgery. Even if your doctor finds a diagnosable issue in an X-ray or MRI, it may not be the underlying cause of the pain. If you choose to go the route of surgery, you may still have ongoing pain after recovery and physical therapy. Then there is the frustration if your doctor finds nothing. Your pain or discomfort seems specific, but there is no explanation or medical reason. This mysterious "nothing" can make you feel a little crazy. I was beside myself when doctors told me that my foot pain was "in my head" and that I should see a psychotherapist. I knew my physical pain was real, even if the doctors didn't have an explanation for it. I was back at square one and very frustrated.

Medical science hasn't found a way to cure chronic conditions—that's why they are chronic. Pain medication can be necessary and useful for pain that is related to acute trauma and disease, but when it is taken in an attempt to resolve pain that falls in the chronic gap of the medical spectrum, the results are usually minimal at best. Pain medication masks the problem *temporarily* and is almost always accompanied by negative consequences like stomach issues or dependence on the medication when taken long term. That's why doctors prescribe pain medication for temporary relief and not indefinitely.

In addition, taking pain medication for long periods of time can drain your body's internal resources, sap your energy, and slow your metabolism. Just as the TV commercials tell you, many pharmaceuticals have unwanted side effects that often create multiple new symptoms. Meanwhile, your body continues to send signals for help—except you can't feel the pain signal anymore. Without the ability to experience pain, you are at risk for greater damage to your joints from repetition and injury. Taking pain medication is like removing the battery out of your kitchen fire alarm when you know that your toaster might catch fire. Turning off the alarm doesn't fix the toaster! Removing the batteries or taking pain medication means your alert system is not going to be able to signal you when you need it most. I have seen countless clients who have chronic pain in their neck, low back, or joints but feel like they've tried everything. After multiple pain medications, cortisone shots, and endless other pain-management interventions, they come to me, still in pain. You may have already learned the hard way that trying to manage pain can be exhausting, expensive, time consuming, and ineffective. Yet, the common belief is that once discomfort and pain become part of your daily life, "managing" it is the only option.

There is no magic pill or shot to heal chronic pain. It's true. Your doctor will likely tell you the same. Medication can't resolve chronic pain because it doesn't address the cause—the repetition of daily living. I don't believe science will ever find a pharmaceutical drug or surgery that will cure the effects of repetition on your connective tissue system. Pain medication is simply the wrong tool for the job.

I understand how it feels when you have pain and all you want is to find someone or something to fix it for you. Realizing that, I want you to think differently about pain as well as your ability to take back control and live pain-free. The MELT Method resolves pain that falls in the chronic gap. If you are healthy and pain-free, MELT will help you stay that way—proactively. If you are recovering from an injury or receiving medical or rehabilitative care, MELT complements this care, and in many cases, improves your results. Beyond pain medication, no matter what your health or level of fitness, you have a new choice with MELT.

▶ Reality Check: Exercise

I love being active, and I do some form of exercise every day. It is easy to grasp why being active is better than being sedentary when it comes to maintaining a healthy life today and tomorrow. However, what I have learned is that exercise and rehabilitation protocols don't resolve pain and discomfort. That's right, functional exercises, stretching, practicing yoga, or even massaging muscles may give you temporary relief, but these activities usually don't provide resolution. That's because the focus on strengthening and stretching muscles is an effort to fix a false problem.

The myth is that if you have joint pain, it's due to muscle imbalance and weakness. The concept is that making muscles stronger and longer will create better alignment and eliminate pain. The truth is, when you have pain, it's not because your muscles are weak. In fact, many of your muscles have to work so hard to compensate for skeletal misalignment that they become overworked and fatigued whether you're moving or not. The connective tissue system, not the muscle system, is responsible for misalignment, imbalance, chronic pain, and discomfort. Once you rehydrate your connective tissue, muscle compensation and imbalance improve and your muscles don't have to work overtime. Then you can exercise in a way that actually improves overall performance, balance, and movement.

If that doesn't fully convince you, consider what I believe is the most closely guarded secret in the fitness industry: almost all professionals in the fitness industry have chronic pain. I first realized this fact when I was seeking a solution for my foot pain. What I found was that most fitness professionals believed that pain was a price you pay for looking great and working in the fitness industry. Once I realized the effects of repetition on my body, it all began to make sense. At the time, I was teaching twenty-eight fitness classes a week. I drank lots of water and ate healthy food, yet I didn't know I was dehydrating myself by neglecting my connective tissue.

Today, the need to care for the connective tissue system is still ignored or misunderstood by most exercise and rehabilitation professionals. The one aspect of the connective tissue system that is sometimes addressed is the myofascia. This is the layer of connective tissue around (and within) all muscles. Myofascial approaches focus on knots, blood flow, and imbalance in muscles by using intense, direct pressure. Although a skilled therapist can make notable changes in muscles using myofascial techniques, the connective tissue system is still not addressed. Without care for the connective tissue as a continuous system, muscle imbalance, misalignment, and pain cannot be resolved.

The reason I can cycle, run, and lift weights on a regular basis without any pain or discomfort is because I MELT. In just minutes, I can undo the negative effects of my active lifestyle so I get all of the positive results and none of the negative side effects. If you aren't currently active because your body doesn't feel good or you don't feel able, MELT can help you turn that around. MELT will help you undo the negative effects of your repetitive positions so you feel better and your body is prepared for activity. I hear again and again that being active is more effortless and enjoyable when you don't have pain. If you are active, even if you are a professional athlete, MELT will reduce the negative effects of your repetitive movements and also improve your performance in multiple ways.

▶ From Problem to Solution

I've solved the puzzle of chronic pain, and I want to share with you what I know. I want you to have an understanding of the systems that are currently unaddressed by medicine and fitness. I want you to understand why it is so important that you take care of your connective tissue and nervous systems—not because I said so, but because it makes sense. When I first learned this information, it blew my mind. I know you will have epiphanies like I did as you learn what's going on in your body and what's been missing from all you've been told about how to care for yourself.

I'm going to teach you how to be your own pain-resolution specialist and address the cause of your pain. MELT is the very first self-care program that rehydrates connective tissue and rebalances the nervous system. This is what allows your body to release long-held tension and discomfort caused by the repetitive postures and movements of everyday living. MELT will also help you reduce accumulated stress in the nervous system, which helps improve your overall health and wellness. When you activate your body's powerful healing mechanisms with MELT, you will experience more than just pain relief. You will open the door to a lifetime of improved health, energy, vitality, and longevity.

Far beyond weight loss and exercise, through a series of easy, precise techniques—using simple, specialized equipment like soft body rollers and small balls—this groundbreaking concept will soon become your missing link to better living. If you are ready to learn the wondrous power of your connective tissue system, take a deep breath and get ready to MELT.

2

The Power of Connective Tissue

I hope you are as excited to learn about the healing and pain-relieving power of connective tissue as I was. I remember clearly the first time I became fully aware of connective tissue. I was at a six-day human cadaver dissection workshop led by theologian, Rolfer, and anatomist Gil Hedley. We were exploring how the body's systems are connected by dissecting cadavers, layer by layer, instead of the traditional way of studying the body's parts separately. After spending three hours carefully removing most of the skin from the body in front of me, I sat back with a blank stare.

"What the heck is that?" I said to Gil.

"It's the superficial fascia," Gil replied in a very matter-of-fact way.

"What is it doing there?" I said with a bewildered look.

"It's the system that supports and protects us," he replied with a mischievous smile. "It's the first layer of the three-dimensional network that gives us our shape and allows us to sense the world around us."

"What do you mean *system*? It's just a part of the skin, right? I mean . . . it's a tissue. Why are you calling it a system? The connective tissue isn't a *system*, is it?"

Gil continued to smile. "Oh my, I think this experience is going to change your life, Sue. This tissue is a continuous, fluid system that connects all other systems of the body and gives them individual space at the same time. In a cadaver we can identify multiple connective tissue layers, but in a living body, this vibrant, fluid-filled tissue creates a seamless, weblike matrix," he said. "Welcome to my world."

Could this fluid system be creating the movement under the skin that I could sense with my hands? I had never heard anyone talk about what I could feel, and suddenly someone was describing it. On an intellectual level, I was blown away and totally intrigued with this new explanation of the connective tissue system. But I have to be honest: emotionally, I was quite angry. How could I have studied the human body in such detail and spent countless hours reading, writing, and even teaching about anatomy only to find that there was a vital system that I had never even heard of? This was the first time I had ever seen the seamless superficial layer. In the many dissections I had done during school, the superficial fascia was tossed in the bucket with the skin so we could study the "good stuff." For a decade I had incorporated what I thought were progressive ideas about myofascia and connective tissue—but only in how it gave muscles their connection and helped in dynamic motion. No one had ever called it a system before. I wanted a refund for all the money I had spent on my higher education. I wanted to call my professors and tell them that what they were teaching was wrong and a disservice to anyone wanting to work with living humans.

After I got over being angry, I needed to know everything about this tissue and how it could scientifically be defined as a system. I needed evidence to back up what Gil had introduced to me in the dissection. I had a burning desire for tangible evidence of why my hands-on techniques were able to yield such extraordinary changes. I was never comfortable with the idea that I had an unexplainable "gift." Like many other bodyworkers, I wanted proof, not just philosophy or belief alone. Suddenly a new door was open for me to learn what this system was and how it related to my hands-on skill.

From 2001 to 2004, I all but disappeared from the fitness education circuit as I dove into the field of fascial research. Soon I had the privilege of meeting researcher Robert Schleip and was somehow welcomed into this budding field of science and research. What I found got me (and kept me) out of pain, changed my career, and put me on the road to creating MELT. I developed new models to explain the connective tissue system. I've since taught hundreds of other fitness and healing professionals the science of MELT, and I watched as this information changed their lives and careers too. The reports they've given me about the lives they've touched has made me profoundly grateful for the gift I received all those years ago in Gil Hedley's workshop.

This information can change your life too. You are about to enter the fascinating world of fascia, where you will uncover your ability to influence your health in ways that you never imagined.

▶ The Fascia-nating World of Fascia

Connective tissue is found everywhere in the body. The particular type of connective tissue I am referring to is scientifically called fascia. Fascia is made up of collagen, elastin, and other fibers that are bathed in cellular fluid. In your connective tissue, there are cells, scientifically referred to as fibroblasts, which are responsible for producing all the fluid and fibrous components of the tissue. Many familiar parts of your body—tendons, ligaments, disks, cartilage, and even the membranes around your brain and organs—are made of fascia. These parts seem separate, yet they are all physically connected and part of the connective tissue system's adaptable, supportive architecture.

Connective tissue surrounds every structure, including bones, organs, muscles, and nerves, and it makes up the fluid environment around every cell. Indeed, every cell in your body relies on this "extracellular matrix" to function properly. This three-dimensional, interactive environment supports and informs cells about the mechanical and biochemical changes around them. The connective tissue fluid permits the transportation of oxygen, nutrients, and waste from cell to cell. It is also the environment in which most of your sensory nerves live and work.

This is a very new area of human science. In the year 2000, an Internet search using the keyword *fascia* yielded only 1,500 results. Today, that number is 51 million and rising rapidly. We know so much more today than we did only fifteen years ago, in part because of the advances in microscopic technology but also because there is dedicated study of connective tissue. Yet there is so much more to be discovered and understood. If you've heard about fascia, you've probably heard about how fascia interacts with muscle (myofascia), not about the health of the connective tissue system as a whole.

In human dissection for medical and academic study, the connective tissue is discarded and disregarded—literally tossed aside with the skin like an irrelevant, accessory tissue covering what are considered the important structures—organs, nerves, muscles, and bones. The outdated view that connective tissue is a passive packing material is still the standard in anatomical texts.

The advancements in fascial research and applications have largely occurred outside of the medical and academic community. The pioneering connective tissue researchers emerged from an unlikely source: manual therapy. Many of them studied directly under Ida Rolf, the founder of the manual therapy technique known as Rolfing. Rolf's desire for her protégés to seek out the scientific explanation for the therapeutic results of her method drives much of the research going on today. Because of the efforts of these Rolfers-turned-researchers (including Fernando Bertolucci, John Cottingham, Steve Evanko, Tom Findley, Gil Hedley, Kai Hodeck, Eric Jacobsen, Tom Myers, Robert Schleip, and Adjo Zorn), we have many answers—and even more questions.

The work of these pioneers expanded and refined my understanding of the connective tissue. Their research gave me a new understanding of its essential properties, multiple functions, and why it is now called a system. I've been able to share their findings, and now, with the completion of the first study focused on MELT, I am only at the beginning of my journey into discovering more about connective tissue, nervous system regulation, and self-care through scientific research.

I've spent years simplifying this complex new science into models and language that anyone can understand and apply to his or her own body. You don't have to understand the molecular components and scientific properties of the connective tissue system in order to care for it. I want you to know the elements of connective tissue that are the most relevant to your health and longevity. I am going to show you how to influence the health and supportiveness of your connective tissue system by directly addressing these elements.

Hydration

How can a fluid system be supportive? Think of a sponge: when it's dry, it's stiff, but when it's moist, it's flexible, adaptable, and resilient. You can twist, squeeze, or compress a moist sponge, and it returns to its original shape. Your body's connective tissue is similar: when it's hydrated, it's buoyant and adaptable. But when it's dehydrated, it gets stiff and inflexible.

Approximately three-quarters of the connective tissue is made up of fluid. The rest is composed of repair cells, filaments, and fibers, such as collagen and elastin, suspended in this fluid. This tissue is the most abundant material in the body, and the health of this tissue relies on hydration. Connective tissue must have enough fluid for its many functions, including responding, adapting, and morphing to provide cushion in joints, space between every cell and organ, and an easy glide between muscles. Of course, when I'm talking about maintaining adequate hydration for this essential system to do its job, I'm not just saying that you need to drink more water. Drinking enough water is an important aspect, but it's just not enough.

Have you ever heard people say that when they drink water, it goes right through them? This means that their body (like a dried-out sponge) cannot properly absorb and use the water—they've become *cellularly* dehydrated. Every cell in the body is at risk of becoming dehydrated due to the lack of fluid in the cell's environment, the connective tissue system. The kidneys can get overstressed from processing the excess, unused fluid. The need to go to the bathroom frequently can deter a person from drinking a healthy amount of water, which in turn accelerates whole body dehydration.

When your cells are chronically dehydrated, drinking all the water in the world won't get that fluid back into your tissues. The dehydrated cells have learned that the surrounding fluid is stagnant and murky, which is often referred to as toxicity in the health care field. Even though the cells desperately need fresh fluid, they'd rather stay thirsty than drink what's available to them. But when you stimulate the connective tissue with MELT, the connective tissue cells can absorb and use the water you drink to produce connective tissue fluid. The new fluid moving in the connective tissue system stimulates all cells of the body to take in the fresh fluid, which extends the life of the cells. What's so amazing about the connective tissue is that you can transform dehydrated tissue into a healthy, hydrated state by using specific, manual techniques. MELT simulates these techniques, and you can do it on your own.

Dehydration

Dehydration of the connective tissue is caused by the repetitive stress and strain of day-to-day living. Your habitual movements and postures—whatever you do most during any given day—create dehydration and joint compression. Repetitive stressors range from sitting at a desk to running a marathon. Carrying children and heavy bags creates stress and compression, as do your sleeping positions and the gentlest forms of exercise. Medication, environmental toxins, poor diet, and sleep habits cause further dehydration in the connective tissue. Dehydration is part of living, so whether you're sedentary or active, young or old, it's happening to you. Exercise, nutrition, meditation, and proper rest are not enough to keep this tissue hydrated over time.

The trouble really begins when dehydrated connective tissue in one area spreads to other areas. The more areas of dehydration there are, the less fluid absorption occurs in the connective tissue system overall, causing dehydration to become a systemic problem—and ultimately, causing body-wide cellular dehydration. Without adequate fluid, the connective tissue loses its ability to be adaptable, supportive, and strong, which affects your joints, muscles, nerves, organs, and every cell of your body.

The progression of dehydration from one area to the whole body can be understood by looking at the connective tissue system like a river. Fluid flows throughout the body at a constant rate and direction. Pockets of dehydration in joints or regions of the body, such as in your knee or low back, are like sediment in the body's river. Water is diverted around the sediment, and over time, the dry area becomes larger, like a sandbar turning into a small island. I have seen this in cadavers even after all the fluid has been removed. These areas of dehydration cause a disruption of continuity and support in the connective tissue system. For example, if you have dehydration in your thumbs from texting, over time that dehydration can spread to the wrist, up the forearm, and into the neck. When you MELT, you erase the negative effects of repetition from your daily activities.

The Ripple Effect of Dehydration

Dehydration in the river of connective tissue affects more than your joints. Remember, every organ, nerve, and cell is also surrounded and supported by this fluid tissue. When chronic dehydration is present, your body has to work harder to maintain the function of its organs and systems.

On a microscopic level, connective tissue dehydration triggers a protective response in cells. Your cells form a seal around themselves to try to preserve the fluid inside when the fluid environment outside is stagnant or lacking. Unfortunately, this means that essential nutrients, minerals, and available fluids are blocked from getting into the cell. Without these necessary cellular building blocks, hormone and enzyme production, cell-to-cell communication, and metabolism are all hindered. This leads to bone and muscle loss, increased fat storage, and premature cell death, all of which accelerate the aging process.

Just as pain acts as a signal that connective tissue dehydration is putting stress on the muscles, joints, and nerves, when your organs and cells lack adequate hydration, they send signals of distress. "Everyday" symptoms—like headaches, sugar cravings, poor sleep, irritability, digestive discomfort, difficulty focusing, or low energy—could be a sign that the connective tissue needs your attention.

The relationship between sleep, concentration, or digestion and the connective tissue may not be obvious, because how symptoms manifest and their intensity vary greatly from person to person. However, when you improve the state of hydration in the connective tissue environment, you may find that these seemingly unrelated symptoms subside. Your body is better able to heal itself when the environment of connective tissue is hydrated and in its optimal state.

▶ We Are Not Robots

Many of us have accepted a very robotic, mechanical view of our body. By mistaking our muscles and bones as the body's structural support system, we've confused muscular strength with structural stability. Our structure is stable because of the sophisticated, three-dimensional architecture that the connective tissue system provides. The connective tissue acts as adaptable, supportive scaffolding for all our parts—protecting the muscles, bones, nerves, and organs so your body can move efficiently without damage.

This aspect of the connective tissue system can be described as a tensegrity model. The word *tensegrity*—a combination of the words *tension* and *integrity*—was coined by architect Buckminster Fuller to describe a structural, oppositional relationship in which an object has the ability to resist distortion of its shape when mechanical stress is applied. Tensegrity structures use minimal energy to maintain their shape because they are stable in all directions, absorb force through all the elements inside their structure, and function independently of gravity.

In the human body, the three-dimensional, seamless network of the connective tissue system is responsible for managing tension and compression in a balanced yet oppositional way. The body's oppositional relationships allow us to remain upright and balanced against gravity with minimal damage or friction to the joints and vital organs. Head-to-toe tensional relationships within the connective tissue dictate the position of our bones and joints at rest and during movement. If the connective tissue is dehydrated, the body's tensegrity declines. When you see rounded shoulders, knock knees, or a bunion, you are seeing outward signs of a lack of tensional integrity. The apparent misalignment and imbalance in each of these examples never occur in isolation. When one joint or region of the body is misaligned, another region shifts out of alignment in the opposing direction so that your body can remain upright. For example, look at someone standing. If the head shifts forward, the ribs shift backward, the hips shift forward, and this pattern continues all the way down to the feet. If this oppositional shifting didn't occur, a forward head position would allow gravity to topple you over.

The ability of the connective tissue to adapt its architecture and temporarily adjust is a good thing and allows the body to maintain an upright position. When your movements are repetitive and these positions are habitual, however, temporary adjustments become chronic misalignments. The body's ability to stay stable and still in one area as muscles move another area is only possible because of this supportive architectural scaffolding.

The extensible quality of connective tissue is an important element of this adaptable, supportive scaffolding. Not to be confused with flexibility, which has to do with muscles, *extensibility* is a term I use to describe the pliable and elastic supportiveness of connective tissue. Although connective tissue does have elastic qualities, it is made to resist stretch so it can manage the balance between tension and compression. Without this quality, muscles would tear and joints would excessively compress. However, muscles can't stretch or contract properly if the surrounding connective tissue has poor extensibility. Extensibility of connective tissue requires hydration. Without hydration, connective tissue loses its ability to support our joints, which causes a chain reaction throughout the entire body. Muscles become overworked and sometimes locked, bones misalign, and joints either compress or become too loose depending on their location within the architecture. Nerve transmission becomes impaired, blood flow becomes restricted, and joints become inflamed.

The connective tissue system will always support whatever position you place your body in with the least amount of effort for as long as it can. That's why you can sit for hours in a slumped position in front of your computer with little effort or pain. However, when the tissue becomes chronically dehydrated in any area, the body's tensional integrity declines, muscle tension picks up the slack, and feelings of discomfort arise.

You can't stretch, strengthen, or will your way into better tensional integrity. The only way to restore the balance between tension and compression is to restore the system responsible for tensegrity architecture—the connective tissue! Rehydrating your connective tissue system with MELT will enable your body to realign itself. When you restore the fluid state of connective tissue, all your joints benefit, your muscles relax, and your body becomes more efficient.

▶ The Body's Brain

Have you ever thought about why it is so easy to carry on a conversation while walking? You take it for granted that you don't have to think about how to move—you just do. How does that work?

It's a widely held belief that movement is created when the brain gives a command through a nerve impulse that tells particular muscles to move a particular body part.

But it's just not that simple. There is far more to movement than the brain telling the muscles to move.

The latest studies about the connective tissue confirm that there is a massive amount of communication occurring within the body with little to no input from your central nervous system or brain. Cell to cell, organ to organ, and joint to joint, this communication is occurring on an electrical and vibrational level through the fluid system of the connective tissue.

At any given moment, there is more information being transmitted through the connective tissue system than there is through the nervous system. Furthermore, the speed of connective tissue communication is more complex and frequently faster. Information is taken in and transmitted through sensory receptors in the tissue, called proprioceptors and mechanoreceptors. This is what I call Body Sense. When your Body Sense is poor, you have to rely more heavily on your five common senses, which can be exhausting and cause you to feel uncoordinated. Proprioceptors detect changes in position, compression, and tension within the body. The mechanorecep-tors' primary role is to sense pressure that is potentially harmful to your body. This pressure can be caused by your movements, which change joint and organ positions, or by forces outside your body, anything from a hug to dropping something on your foot. When you have chronic misalignment, the proprioceptors and mechanoreceptors alert the brain to potential damage through the sensory nerves and you feel pain. These sensory receptors were believed to be exclusively in the muscle system, yet new science has revealed that there are *billions more* in the connective tissue system. These discoveries radically change how we view communication within the body and the origin of pain.

Another mind-blowing concept is that the connective tissue system receives more information from outside the body than the brain does through the five common senses. Indeed, fascial researcher Robert Schleip calls the connective tissue the largest sensory organ in the body. Just as the receptors in the connective tissue pick up changes in position, movement, weight, and pressure from inside the body, they also take in that information from outside the body. Your body is constantly using this information without your conscious awareness to regulate joint position, posture, and stability. Consider what occurs when there's a sudden change in the pavement beneath you, or you unknowingly step from concrete to grass or from curb to street. If you had to rely solely on your eyes to tell your brain to signal your muscles to remain upright, you would lose your balance and fall—all the time. Instead, information about the change underfoot is picked up by the sensory receptors in the connective tissue before you ever step on your foot. The connective tissue system has already started to adjust and modify every single joint in your body in relationship to gravity so you don't damage your organs or joints and you don't fall. Your brain gets involved *after* this massive relay has already occurred.

Although the brain does direct muscles, it cannot do this properly without the information it receives about the musculoskeletal system from the sensory receptors living in the connective tissue. Before the brain signals your muscles to move, the connective tissue system prepares your body by creating tensegrity to minimize friction and compression in joints. In order to align and stabilize the joints, connective tissue creates what's called "pre-anticipatory tensional stress" between joints. This act of body-wide pre-stressing lets the brain know how much motor nerve impulse to send so the muscles can create the proper leverage, contraction, and timing. This supportive tension is what allows your body to remain balanced as you perform any movement, from throwing a baseball to picking up a pen.

Consider the action of jumping. The connective tissue acts as a whole body stabilizing system that regulates your body weight as you push off, float in the air, and then land. The sensors in the connective tissue monitor and support every joint so you can land on your feet without twisting your ankle or tearing a tendon. This protective, supportive response occurs without your having to think about it—so long as the connective tissue system is adequately hydrated.

Every aspect of movement works better when the connective tissue is a hydrated, stable environment for the sensory nerves. Without adequate hydration, internal body communication cannot travel with the necessary speed or accuracy, and sensory nerve transmission and reception becomes disrupted. Without precise information about the body's position, muscle contraction becomes delayed or inhibited—seemingly "weak"—and compensation develops as uninhibited muscles step up to take over. The weakness is not a matter of muscle strength. Instead, it is caused by the lack of accurate neurological communication getting to the right muscle groups at the right time. Movement becomes stiff, labored, and inefficient. Over time, these labored movements become chronic patterns, all of which can occur prior to any discomfort or pain.

It's easy to blame these changes on aging. But in fact, getting older just means you've had more time to accumulate the results of chronic dehydration. Because connective tissue dehydration, not aging, is the root cause of many of these negative effects, you can take action to reverse these symptoms. When you rehydrate your connective tissue, your body's communication, stability, and mobility instantly improve.

▶ The Inflammation Problem

When you think about being inflamed, you may think about bumps and bruises, puffy eyes, or heat and redness on your skin. Although you might recognize these symptoms, do you know what inflammation is or why it happens?

Acute inflammation is an exquisitely complex and powerful aspect of the repair and healing process. When trauma occurs to the body, your immune system dispatches an abundance of repair cells, chemicals, blood, and other fluids to protect and heal the damaged tissue. The inflammation—redness, swelling, stiffness, and heat—is a by-product of this immediate immune response. You experience acute inflammation when you twist your ankle, bump your head, cut or burn yourself, or are stung by a bee. You also experience inflammation when you drink too much alcohol or eat food that your body can't adequately digest. This biological "take control and protect" reaction is a brilliant immune response.

However, there is a different type of inflammation that might be damaging your joints right now, without your even realizing it. This is chronic inflammation, and it can affect you at any age regardless of your lifestyle. Unlike acute inflammation, the swelling, stiffness, and heat are so subtle that you don't even realize they are happening. This subtlety is why chronic inflammation is referred to as low-level or low-grade inflammation. Chronic connective tissue dehydration, joint misalignment, and inflammation go hand in hand. When the connective tissue has regions of dehydration, the tensional architecture is compromised and the joints become chronically misaligned in order to keep you upright and stable. Misaligned joints lose space and their ability to absorb shock. This makes joints susceptible to excess compression, friction, and tension whether you are moving or not. Like scratching a scab over and over, continued repetition doesn't allow the connective tissue in and around joints to rehydrate or repair. This causes a complex biomechanical and chemical chain reaction, one of the results of which is low-level, chronic inflammation. All of this occurs and you don't even realize it. As I always say, this is the blessing and the curse of your body's brilliant design. Because you don't notice the multitude of misalignments, the negative effects of dehydration and inflammation occur without you realizing it.

Eventually chronic inflammation and joint compression escalate and cause noticeable symptoms to arise. You feel stiffness, tenderness, swelling, aching, and even pain. By the time you notice symptoms of chronic inflammation in one joint or area of your body, there are other areas that have chronic joint misalignment, connective tissue dehydration, and inflammation. When you adjust your position, rub the area, crack your joints, or stretch, it doesn't provide long-term relief. As your tensional architecture and posture decline, other parts of your body are affected and more symptoms arise. Nerves are compressed, which can cause tingling, numbness, and pain. Muscles become fatigued, strained, and out of balance, which can cause soreness, inflexibility, and pain. Your risk of injury increases as connective tissue dehydration spreads and nerve transmission declines.

Studies such as those done at the Stanford University School of Medicine show that chronic inflammation, not compression or wear and tear, is the primary cause of joint damage. Chronically inflamed tissues in and around the joints are overheated, stiff, and swollen with stagnant chemicals and fluids. The accumulation of these stagnant fluids damages joints, bones, nerves, tendons, cartilage, and ligaments. I want you to know about chronic inflammation because, according to the Centers for Disease Control and Prevention, 50 percent of people will develop degenerative joint disease, or osteoarthritis, during their lifetime. The CDC also reports that osteoarthritis is the leading cause of chronic disability in the United States. Current medical treatments don't address the root cause, and joint replacement becomes almost inevitable. And chronic inflammation doesn't just damage joints—it also wreaks havoc on your immune system and other aspects of your health, dramatically accelerating the aging process.

MELT helps stop chronic inflammation and can even reverse many of its effects! When you rehydrate connective tissue with MELT, you address connective tissue dehydration and inflammation. You don't have to figure out where you have joint misalignment or compression. When you treat the connective tissue as a system, the tensional architecture of your whole body naturally restores better alignment. When your connective tissue system is hydrated, it can efficiently manage tension and compression every day.

I have seen many people dramatically improve their arthritis symptoms and become active again by using MELT. And if you don't have chronic inflammation, MELT keeps it from occurring. You can keep your joints free of inflammation and help your body's natural healing capabilities stay in optimal condition at any age.

▶ The Good News

Connective tissue dehydration—even chronic cellular dehydration and inflammation— doesn't have to be permanent. The connective tissue is a remarkable, renewable resource. The hydration of the connective tissue can be restored to improve whole body communication, rejuvenate buoyancy and adaptability, and realign joints and posture. New science shows that specific kinds of pressure and pull on connective tissue can be used to create whole body rehydration. This means that rehydrating the connective tissue system requires direct, manual intervention—or, in the case of MELT, stimulation that simulates the effects and results of manual therapy. To wake up the tissues and stimulate them to produce and absorb fresh fluid requires just the right touch. Like squeezing out a sponge so it can then draw in fresh fluid, you can relieve joint compression by applying appropriate compression to the surrounding connective tissue.

To achieve and maintain a healthy, hydrated body, the key is maintenance. The tissue needs regular treatment using MELT or other bodywork as well as consistent water intake. Drink small amounts throughout the day, starting right after you wake up. As you begin to MELT and focus on the consistency of your water intake, you will help the connective tissue absorb this fluid and transport it to other cells. By hydrating your connective tissue, you give yourself the capacity for healing and good health—when the connective tissue is hydrated, the body functions at a more optimal level. Your movements require less effort. You can easily hop up a flight of stairs, get into and out of a chair, and get down to and up from the floor without a thought. You can breathe with ease and sleep well. You feel vibrant, energetic, and clearheaded. Digestion and elimination are easy. Your skin looks bright and supple. You are more likely to experience youthful good health.

Rehydrating your connective tissue—that is, MELTing—can have a powerful effect on your entire body. After following the MELT plan for just a few weeks, you may feel better than you have felt in years—you may even feel better than you ever have. Following the MELT program puts the power to change your body and your life at your fingertips.

3

The Missing Link

As my private practice became transformed by MELT, my clients were experiencing amazing results rehydrating their own connective tissue. They were excited and wanted to learn more. So in 2004, I brought my clients together in one room at a club where I taught indoor cycling and strength classes.

I was so eager to share everything I had learned that I often spent more time talking about the science than teaching the technique. I even brought in strips of cow fascia for show-and-tell. Word quickly spread that I was teaching how to successfully self-treat pain, and soon other people joined the class. I was ecstatic. I went from being the go-to girl for a sweat-filled, muscle-building workout to being a pioneer of pain-free living and longevity.

About a year later, one of the women in my class said, "Sue, I usually have a hard time falling asleep, and I wake up in the middle of the night. Since I've been taking this class, I go to sleep easier and stay asleep longer. Do you think MELT could be helping me sleep better?"

Before I could answer, another woman said, "You know, I've been sleeping better too. I usually have to get up at night to go to the bathroom. Lately I've been sleeping through the night, and I haven't been able to figure out why. Maybe this is it!"

A third woman said, "I have asthma, and I haven't been using my inhaler nearly as much as usual. I definitely think it's this class."

I couldn't stop thinking about what each woman said. I get results with these types of chronic issues using hands-on neurological techniques in my private practice. Yet those techniques are very different from what I was teaching here. The next day in a different class, I asked if anyone had seen benefits other than improvements in pain and physical performance. Everybody started talking at once, sharing all of these amazing improvements:

"I haven't been getting heartburn as much."

"I don't feel like I need a nap in the afternoon."

"My sinus headaches are gone."

"My menstrual cramps have become almost nonexistent."

"My husband said my mood is better and that I seem to be more relaxed."

One woman even said, "MELT is changing my life."

I was blown away. The list of things that people felt MELT was helping with was staggering. What was happening?

The techniques I was teaching focused on rehydrating the connective tissue system. Yet the common thread of the changes they described was improvement in the body's efficiency, which is regulated by the *nervous system.* I could make these kinds of changes one-on-one, but that's not what I was trying to do. Had I unknowingly created a technique that simulates the neurological changes I could make with my hands?

At the time I thought that the connective tissue system and the nervous system were as separate as the digestive system and the skeletal system. There was no research that connected the two. How were these connective tissue techniques helping nervous system regulation? My first theory was that by rehydrating connective tissue, we were improving emotional postures as well as repetitive postures. Tension-filled emotions—such as fear, anger, and grief—give rise to certain visible postures, patterns, and movements. When body language becomes chronic, it causes connective tissue dehydration in the same way that daily repetitive patterns do.

Students in my classes had become more upbeat, energetic, and open. Their faces and shoulders looked relaxed. They seemed to have more of a bounce in their step. It was apparent that their mood and body language were improving. However, erasing emotional postures did not explain how rehydrating connective tissue was improving sleep, digestion, and asthma. There was clearly more going on. Their nervous systems were doing a better job of regulating these functions.

▶ Your Regulators Run the Show

Ask ten neuroscientists how the nervous system manages stress or regulates good health and you'll likely get ten different explanations. What recent science has shown is that the important aspects of the nervous system that influence stress accumulation and its effect on good health are operating outside of your brain's control. Although you can think about how well you slept last night, how fast your heart is beating, when you last had a bowel movement, or how sluggish your metabolism seems, you can't control these functions with your thoughts. It's a good thing that you don't have to think about the five hundred functions of your liver, how often you need to blink, or when food is ready to move from your stomach to your intestines. This is more than your thinking self could process. Instead, all involuntary or automatic functions are regulated in the body by the autonomic nervous system through a sophisticated chemical, electrical, and hormonal orchestration.

There are three subsystems of the autonomic nervous system that are scientifically referred to as the sympathetic, parasympathetic, and the more recently recognized enteric nervous systems. I call this trio of regulators the stress, restore, and gut regulators. When one regulator is out of balance, it affects the other two and causes symptoms to arise. You can't think your way into better function and out of symptoms. What you can do is influence the balance of the autonomic nervous system regulators so your body functions more efficiently and chronic symptoms decrease—if you know how.

MELT is the tool to accomplish this. I want you to know the aspects of your nervous system that MELT is rebalancing so you know why it works. I have simplified my scientific knowledge and empirical understanding of your body's regulation system so you can learn why the MELT techniques can transform your health beyond the elimination of chronic pain.

The stress and restore regulators operate like a seesaw. Together they help the body maintain internal balance by fine-tuning most of the body's vital functions. This give-and-take is happening all the time, without your awareness or control. Traditionally, the stress regulator is referred to as the fight, flight, or freeze response because this regulator goes into overdrive during acute stress. If you needed to get out of the way of an oncoming car, the stress regulator would sharply boost adrenaline and bodily functions such as heart rate, perspiration, breathing, and pupil dilation. Once you are safe, it's the restore regulator that adjusts and normalizes these same functions to bring the body back into balance.

I have come to realize that a broad range of circumstances can trigger the stress regulator—not just acute or traumatic stress. The stress regulator responds to any incoming information, such as driving a car, exercising, walking up stairs, watching TV, taking a bath, having a conversation, gardening, crossing the street, or learning. Each of these activities requires micro-adjustments to your internal systems. This seesaw effect occurs without your conscious control.

Although "stress" is often seen as something that should be alleviated or avoided, stress itself isn't necessarily bad. Your body sees stress as information or movement that requires a response. The restore regulator responds to the stress regulator adjustments by bringing the body back into balance and initiating repair when necessary. The stress and restore regulators are continuously responding and reacting by making countless micro-adjustments twenty-four hours a day. The stress regulator is dominant primarily during your waking hours, and the restore regulator is dominant primarily during sleep. In fact, most of your body's healing and repair take place while you're asleep, although the restore regulator also oversees repair and healing on a smaller scale during your waking hours.

One of the most important tools for a fresh, vibrant, youthful appearance and energy is adequate sleep. During REM (rapid eye movement) sleep, the restore regulator is busy monitoring organ healing, chemical and hormonal balance, and cellular repair.

The enteric nervous system—the third, lesser-known autonomic nervous system regulator, which I call the gut regulator—directly manages every aspect of the gut and digestion. The fact that your body can process whatever you put in it is remarkable. Digestion is a mechanical, chemical, and absorptive process that relies heavily on fluid. Fluid allows food to be digested, nutrients to be absorbed and transported into the bloodstream, and waste to move through and leave the body. This highly intricate system has more parts than the transmission of a car. The gut regulator receives little intervention from the brain. Instead, the connective tissue system provides a network for organ-to-organ communication. Like the brain, the gut has its own neurotransmitters. In fact, there are more neurotransmitters in the gut than in the brain. The gut also produces chemicals and hormones such as serotonin, adrenaline, and testosterone, which are used by all three regulators.

Regulation Efficiency

If your autonomic nervous system regulation is operating efficiently, all the regulators do their jobs with minimal effort. Your regulators ebb and flow, each getting its time to be dominant and to regulate your body's functions as needed. The restore regulator supports your ability to fall asleep, stay asleep, and wake up rested. While sleeping, your body repairs itself. Your gut regulator manages your digestion, and as a result you can eliminate without difficulty. Your stress regulator responds appropriately to each instance of incoming stress, and your restore regulator returns your body to equilibrium.

In this efficient state, the seesaw always returns to balance with minimal energy. Your energy is good throughout the day, and you can handle difficult situations with ease. Further, your regulators constantly make adjustments to bring you back to balance even when you challenge them by doing things like eating processed foods, drinking too much alcohol, experiencing a difficult situation, sitting all day, or not getting enough sleep. If these challenges occur for a day or so, your regulators can efficiently bring you back to balance without signs, symptoms, or your conscious awareness. Wouldn't it be nice to be in this state all the time?

Regulation Inefficiency

These challenges, over time, inhibit the regulators' ability to efficiently bring you back to balance. You also challenge your regulators when you don't allow each one its time to be dominant. If you have a full stomach when you exercise or go to bed, or if you keep working when you're completely exhausted, none of your regulators can do their job well.

Consider some of the activities you do to relieve the stress of the day—consuming caffeine, eating sugary foods or a heavy meal, drinking alcohol, using recreational drugs, and endlessly watching TV or surfing the Internet. When you do these activities too close to bedtime, they keep your stress regulator active when you need it to be winding down. While you are sleeping, light, noise, pets, kids, and other disturbances keep the restore regulator from its time to be dominant and oversee repair. The regulators are so connected that when one is being constantly challenged, the relationship among all the regulators becomes imbalanced. If you don't get a good night's sleep, the restore regulator can't do its job of repairing the complex gut system. This leads to gut distress day after day, which interferes with your ability to have sound, restorative sleep. A high-stress work and home environment or always "burning the candle at both ends" creates overactivity in the stress regulator, which affects your gut and the quality of your sleep.

It can't be stated enough: restorative sleep is paramount. If the restore regulator doesn't have enough time or fluid to fully repair, replenish, and heal, you start the next day with a backlog of accumulated stress. Over time the entire regulation system becomes inefficient. Regulation inefficiency itself constantly activates the stress regulator, taking you further out of balance. This inefficient state requires more effort and energy, and your autonomic ability to adapt and respond declines. Your organs, muscles, brain, connective tissue, and regulators are working harder, even when you're not doing anything. It's like stepping on the gas when your car is in neutral. This slowly exhausts every system of your body and your body's resources, all before you even know it is happening. Your regulation system has to prioritize which functions get attention and energy, and it opts to monitor your vital functions, such as heart rate and breathing, instead of hair growth and muscle repair. This makes you look older and feel exhausted.

This prioritization is a protective mode to ensure that the regulators have enough energy and fluid to monitor and repair your vital functions. It's like your computer giving you a message that it must operate in safety mode. Your computer doesn't shut down, it just runs slowly and you don't have access to all of your programs. Unlike your computer, however, you don't realize that this protective mode is occurring, and initially there aren't any warning signs or symptoms. Common occurrences such as uncontrollable yawning in the afternoon, gas or heartburn, cloudy-headedness, bloat, dry skin or hair, anxiety, and tired muscles when you exercise can all be signs of regulation inefficiency. These are your subtle signals. If you rehydrate your connective tissue when you first notice these symptoms, you can turn them around in a short period of time.

We usually view these symptoms as normal and temporary inconveniences and move on. Meanwhile, when your regulation is in protective mode, your gut isn't processing food or eliminating efficiently, and your cellular repair is slow. These slowdowns cause excess waste to build up in the body. Your body must store this waste somewhere—and that "somewhere" is your connective tissue. As waste gets dumped into the connective tissue system, it collects like sediment, causing the connective tissue to become stagnant and dehydrated.

Stuck Stress

I call this stagnation and dehydrated connective tissue stuck stress. Stuck stress accumulates, which causes the fluid flow and supportive environment of the connective tissue system to decline further. And just as inadequate fluid creates a negative chain reaction in the gut, rehydration of your connective tissue can restore your gut's ability to efficiently work to fuel your body so you have the energy to do the things you love. Rehydration can turn around your repair system as well. Having enough fluid in your connective tissue is vital for both the quality of your sleep and daily repair. Your capacity for repair and healing is completely reliant on all of your cells' ability to take in healthy fluid and nutrients and emit waste. When the environment around your cells is stagnant, cell walls seal themselves off and resist absorption. This makes cell renewal impossible—instead of renewing, the cells die.

Cell renewal is what keeps you looking and feeling young. Without adequate absorption of nutrients and fluid, cells can't renew, and signs of aging such as wrinkles, age spots, and sagging skin occur. However, the damaging effects go far beyond appearance. Slow cell renewal accelerates bone and muscle loss, impairs organ function, impedes immune response, and slows metabolism. I have seen rehydration improve these circumstances in people of all ages and states of health.

What I have discovered is that the relationship between the regulators and the connective tissue system is as closely linked as the relationship between the regulators themselves. When the regulators are imbalanced, the connective tissue system is dehydrated, and the opposite is also true. It doesn't matter which comes first—stuck stress or regulation inefficiency—they always coexist. Nor does it matter if the catalyst was part of a healthy or unhealthy lifestyle, activity or inactivity. This happens to everyone because we haven't known that we could rebalance the regulators and rehydrate the connective tissue. I am going to show you easy, effective ways to do both.

The cause of stuck stress accumulation is daily living. The contributing factors—repetitive movements, habitual and emotional postures, emotional and gut distress, and poor or inhibited body communication—are happening to all of us throughout our lives.

If we don't address the causes, our body's inefficiency escalates and our stuck stress accumulates. Symptoms that used to come and go now become chronic or a greater annoyance. You may find yourself with symptoms like weight gain, low libido, chronic constipation, headaches, fatigue, low back pain, eczema, anxiety, and insomnia. By the time you have these symptoms, there's a significant underlying problem—but all you want is relief. You may find relief of individual symptoms through medication. But wouldn't you know it—this temporary chemical alteration causes further regulation imbalance and ultimately makes the problem worse. Now you can learn to reduce stuck stress and help your regulators return to a balanced state.

Your Body's Stability System

The Autopilot is what I call the link between your connective tissue and nervous systems, and it regulates and stabilizes all other systems of the body without your conscious control. The Autopilot is a receptive, regulating system of support, protection, stability, and body communication. One of the functions that the Autopilot oversees is your body's balance and stability during movement and at rest. The Autopilot does this for you every second of every day without your having to think about it.

Instead of trying to explain all of this complex science, let me use this analogy: To regulate your body's stability, the Autopilot works like a global positioning system, or GPS. A GPS uses radio wave signals sent from satellites to determine its location. The GPS must have an unobstructed connection to multiple satellites in order to provide accurate position information.

Like a GPS, your Autopilot is always trying to find your body's center of gravity, which is in the center of your pelvis. The joints of your body are the satellites, and Body Sense is the radio wave signals. Ideally, there is a continuous signal relay from your feet, head, fingers, and every joint in between to your pelvis, so your body knows where it is in relationship to the ground. This allows your Autopilot to keep your body balanced and support and protect your organs, nerves, bones, and joints. This relay should be happening all the time whether you are moving, sitting, or even sleeping. If there is static in the signal, or a poor connection, from dehydration or inflammation in the connective tissue, your Autopilot must compensate to keep your body upright. This inefficient, protective mode occurs without your realizing it.

▶ The Solution

Why is MELT so effective in eliminating the body of stuck stress? It is my theory that MELT rebalances the regulators by influencing your restore regulator to become dominant while you are awake. Then, when you sleep, your restore regulator can work more efficiently and do its job to repair and heal your body. Rebalancing the stress and restore regulators naturally brings the gut regulator back into balance and improves overall regulation.

My clients were seeing their symptoms disappear because they were finally addressing the fundamental cause of their symptoms, not just trying to mask them. By rehydrating the connective tissue, we helped to reduce the amount of stress in the nervous system overall, which improved the nervous system's ability to regulate itself. That's the brilliance of the body. When your body gets the support it needs, it heals itself. MELT rebalances the regulators and rehydrates the fluid environment that all body systems rely on. And MELT will do this for you too.

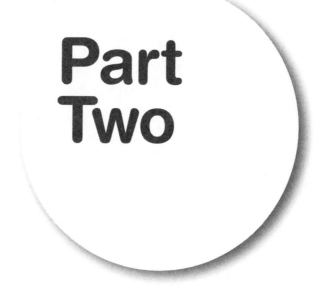

Part Two

4

Becoming a Hands-Off Bodyworker

Your life, and your body, is full of stress—stuck stress. You know this already, because you have seen firsthand how stress has manifested in your body. The impulse, when you understand this, is to try to reduce, eliminate, combat, or manage stress in your life. But this doesn't work—you know that. Now you are going to learn that the key to getting rid of pain and fatigue lies in a different direction. At the core of your recovery is the ability to rid your body of stuck stress.

It doesn't matter how or why the stuck stress got there. Repetitive movements and postures, anxiety, poor sleep or diet, sedentary lifestyle, or life circumstances such as aging, trauma, pregnancy, and surgery all have the same effect on the neurofascial system: the accumulation of stuck stress. When stress accumulation occurs, your Autopilot gets knocked out of what I call the Efficiency Zone, or EZ Zone, and your whole body becomes inefficient in seemingly undetectable ways. Over time the daily repair and healing that occurs primarily while you sleep declines. You may have no idea that your body is operating inefficiently until you notice a symptom.

I have found that before pain, symptoms, or even whole body inefficiency occurs, there are four systemic effects of the accumulation of stuck stress in your neurofascial system.

Connective Tissue Dehydration: Pockets or areas of dehydration in joints or regions of the body

Compression: A loss of joint space in the neck and/or low back

NeuroCore Imbalance: Imbalance in the mechanism I call the NeuroCore, which is responsible for whole body stabilization and grounding and for the protection of vital organs

Faulty Body Sense: Inaccurate signaling in your involuntary body-wide communication system, or what I call Body Sense, which is required for efficient movement and balance

These four effects make it impossible for your Autopilot to remain in the EZ Zone, and they occur without your realizing it. The consequence is that your whole body becomes inefficient, which interferes with your body's ability to repair, adjust, and heal on a daily basis. This inability to repair is what fundamentally causes symptoms to appear.

Symptoms may include:

- Stiffness and achiness upon rising
- Inflammation
- Trouble sleeping
- Constipation
- Extra weight
- Lack of energy
- Stress injuries
- Joint pain or swelling
- Headaches
- Bloating
- Poor digestion
- Wrinkles
- Cellulite
- Being prone to accidents
- Poor posture
- Poor balance
- Protruding low belly
- Uncoordinated movement
- Difficulty sitting for long periods
- Fidgetiness
- Leg cramps
- Restless legs
- Stiff, tight muscles
- Loose, hypermobile joints
- Brain fog
- Anxiety
- Depression
- Concentration issues
- Mood swings

If you recognize any of these symptoms, I want you to start looking at them in a new way. Your symptoms are a signal that stuck stress has accumulated, you are out of the

EZ Zone, and your Autopilot is operating inefficiently. Symptoms that may seem unrelated—such as constipation, back pain, and headaches—are all connected by their underlying cause: stuck stress. When you address the accumulation of stuck stress, your symptoms will improve or go away.

You must be in the EZ Zone to eliminate symptoms and pain. You can't just exercise, diet, supplement, meditate, surgically repair, or medicate yourself and then become pain- or symptom-free. You can't think your way out of stuck stress and back into the EZ Zone (in case you were thinking you could). Focusing on masking your pain or curing your symptoms provides only short-term relief, further exhausts your body, and causes more stuck stress to accumulate. I want you to shift your focus away from pain and any other symptoms you're experiencing. With MELT and your understanding of your body's desire to return to the EZ Zone, you will experience immediate changes in your body. Your body's daily repair and healing mechanisms will be able to make long-term improvements to your chronic pain and other symptoms in ways that were not possible before. One of the best things about MELT is that you will be able to sense the changes right away *and* every time you MELT.

▶ The Four R's

MELT directly addresses the four effects of stuck stress with the Four R's: Reconnect, Rebalance, Rehydrate, and Release. The Four R's are the MELT formula of self-treatment. Within each category, there are different techniques used to achieve the desired result. The Four R's are the recipe for the most immediate, lasting changes, which is why you will always use all Four R's every time you MELT.

Reconnect techniques heighten Body Sense and the mind-body connection, which is a vital component of your body's daily repair and healing function. You will learn how to use Body Sense, not your common senses, to identify stuck stress and inefficiency and to track your progress. Reconnect techniques also help the Autopilot reacquire its connection to your center of gravity to improve whole-body balance.

Rebalance techniques directly address the NeuroCore stabilizing mechanisms your Autopilot uses to improve balance, grounding, and organ support. Rebalance techniques are subtle yet profound in the changes they create.

Rehydrate techniques restore the fluid state of the connective tissue system. These techniques improve the environment for all your joints, muscles, organs, bones, and cells as well as the tensional integrity of the body. These techniques also decrease inflammation in the joints and improve the fluid and nutrient absorption of every cell.

Release techniques decompress your neck, low back, and the joints of your spine, hands, and feet. Regaining and maintaining the space in your joints will keep you youthful, mobile, and pain-free.

Each R of MELT addresses aspects of all four effects of stuck stress—connective tissue dehydration, compression, NeuroCore imbalance, and faulty Body Sense. You don't need to be an expert on the science of connective tissue and the nervous system to MELT. You don't even need to know what manual therapy is. You just need the Four R's of MELT.

Because connective tissue is one seamless interconnected system that wraps around every muscle, bone, joint, and organ, you can create changes in your whole body, regardless of which technique you are doing or the area you are self-treating. MELT directly affects the systems of the body that no self-care or medical-care modality is able to reach. Before MELT, these results were only available through ongoing, costly therapies from multiple practitioners in a variety of fields, such as acupuncture, structural integration, massage, osteopathy, and craniosacral therapy. With MELT you are the one in charge of rehydrating your connective tissue and rebalancing your nervous system. This makes MELT different from anything previously available.

I have incorporated the multiple modalities that I use in my private practice into the MELT self-treatment techniques. Most of the MELT language, concepts, and philosophies are born out of the traditions of manual therapy, or hands-on bodywork, including Leon Chaitow's and Judith DeLany's Neuromuscular Therapy, John Upledger's CranioSacral Therapy, Ida Rolf's Structural Integration, Bruno Chikly's Lymph Drainage Therapy, and Jean-Pierre Barral's Visceral Manipulation. I am going to teach you how to be your own Hands-Off Bodyworker. Now you are in control. Think of it—you can create immediate changes and feel better in only ten minutes a day. It's that simple. You can unload the accumulated stress in your body so you can feel better today and handle the stress that will inevitably crop up tomorrow. The changes that you will create in your body will radically change your view of how much you can do on your own to become healthy and pain-free. No longer will you have to wait for a symptom or an ache to care for the imbalances and inefficiencies that happen to all of us.

I'm excited for you to sense powerful, immediate changes in your innate balance and alignment. This is one of the first ways you'll know that you are on your way to the life-changing results that occur from incorporating MELT into your regular routine. Here are some other changes you may notice in the first few days or weeks:

- Your body will be much more comfortable during your day-to-day activities.

- Movement will become more effortless and you will feel more stable and flexible.

- You will feel more grounded and clear-minded.

- You will fall asleep more easily and sleep more soundly.

- You will wake up more rested and have more energy throughout your day.

- You will have fewer aches and less pain as well as a greater sense of overall well-being.

As you continue to MELT, you'll regain balance in the nervous system regulators and restore the fluid state of the connective tissue system. This is what will get your Autopilot back to the EZ Zone so daily repair and healing can occur. This usually takes two to three weeks, but for some people it may take as little as a few days, and for others it takes months. It all depends on how much stuck stress your body needs to process. I am going to ask you to try MELT for at least one month to allow your natural healing mechanism to come back online. I will outline your self-treatment plan in the following chapters.

Regardless of your current state of health, MELT helps your body return to a better place. You can MELT every day, but don't be impatient with your body's healing process. If you try to rush it, you will put additional stress on your body, which works against its ability to heal. Whether you MELT every day, every other day, or three times a week, you will be heightening your body's daily repair and healing function. Once you wake up your body's ability to heal, you will have less stuck stress and pain to manage. Your daily repair function can then go to work on other symptoms. How quickly symptoms subside varies for each individual because your collection of symptoms and your history are unique. The reduction in the intensity or frequency of your symptoms will be a gauge for how well your repair and healing function is operating and how often you need to MELT.

MELT is not a cure for symptoms or illness. MELT supports your body's ability to heal itself. The ultimate goal is for you to shift from reacting to your pain and other issues toward proactively using MELT to live a healthy, active, pain-free life.

▶ The Method of MELTing

The method of MELTing is simple—all you need to know is the language of Hands-Off Bodywork. The most basic element of MELTing is the MELT move. A move applies techniques from one of the Four R's to a body part or area of the body using a soft roller. A sequence is a structured progression of MELT moves from two or more of the Four R's that yields a specific result. Before and after any MELT sequence, you will Reconnect to self-assess your results. Reconnecting allows you and your body to identify the immediate changes you've made from the Rebalance, Rehydrate, and Release techniques and encourages you to keep MELTing. Reconnecting before and after is integral to creating lasting changes with MELT.

MELT maps combine a series of sequences to create a complete self-treatment that includes all Four R's: Reconnect, Rebalance, Rehydrate, and Release. This means that every time you MELT, you're addressing all four effects of stuck stress so you can get your Autopilot in the EZ Zone. The MELT Hand and Foot Treatment is a global self-treatment. It applies techniques from all Four R's to the hands and feet using a small ball. The Hand and Foot Treatment can be done on its own or as part of a MELT map.

In Chapters 5 through 9 you will learn the intention and techniques of each R as well as the Hand and Foot Treatment. In each of these chapters, you will have the opportunity to try a few of the moves as you learn about Reconnecting, Rebalancing, Rehydrating, and Releasing. In the next part of the book you will begin your MELT practice by learning the sequences one at a time. You are on your way to becoming a Hands-Off Bodyworker, making lasting changes to your body with the Four R's and getting into the EZ Zone.

5

Reconnect

In this chapter you will learn how powerful it is to reconnect with your body, something you may have felt disconnected from for years. When you are in pain, the tendency is to do anything you can to tune it out or to take a pill to decrease the unpleasant feelings you sense. However, self-awareness is essential to alleviating chronic pain, and it's missing from most, if not all, methods of treating chronic pain.

Learning how to identify where stuck stress is accumulating in your body is an important element in becoming a Hands-Off Bodyworker. Assessment using Reconnect moves is the first step to eliminating chronic pain and improving the way your body functions. Sensing improvements is key to creating lasting changes. Reconnect moves also help your Autopilot reacquire its connection to your center of gravity to boost whole-body balance.

We will start with the Rest Assess. This is the same self-assessment you will be using whenever you MELT, and you will usually conduct it with your eyes closed. This first time, however, you can go through it with your eyes open as you read the following instructions.

To do this assessment, you are going to use your body's internal awareness, or what I call Body Sense. Body Sense is the ability to sense your body's position in relationship to your surroundings. It is the overlooked sixth sense that is as important as the other five. When you do this assessment, use your Body Sense to get a sense of what you feel rather than touching your body, looking at yourself, fidgeting, or adjusting your body's position.

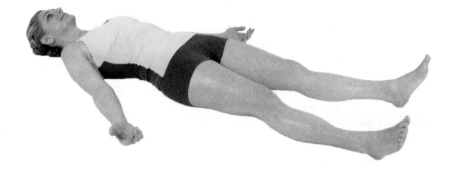

Rest Assess

▶ *Lie on the floor with your arms and legs extended and relaxed, palms face up. Breathe and allow your body to rest on the floor.*

▶ *Notice that there are areas of your body that touch the floor and others that don't. Sense how your body makes a wave formation, alternating between areas that are weighted to the floor (like your head) and others that are off the floor (like your neck), all the way down to your feet. Your sense of this is heightened when your eyes are closed and you only use your Body Sense.*

▶ *Once you sense the areas of your body that are on and off the floor, I want you to gain a sense of the right and left sides of your body. Imagine dividing yourself into a left and right half from head to toe. Notice if one side of your body feels more weighted on the floor or if you sense that one leg feels longer than the other. Remember, don't adjust your body position or look at yourself. By using your internal awareness, you will learn to heighten your Body Sense, which is required for all MELT self-assessments. If you're not sure what you feel, make a mental note of that. That's not uncommon, and I will explain why later.*

▶ *Now try sensing your body with your eyes closed. Remember, feel the wave formation of weighted and nonweighted regions of your body, and notice if one side of your body feels heavier or longer than the other. If you feel like your body is uneven from left to right, you are gaining a sense of what it feels like when you have inefficiency in your Autopilot.*

Remember, one of the functions of the Autopilot is to regulate your body's balance and stability during movement and rest. When you assessed yourself, if you felt heavier on one side or if one leg felt longer than the other, your Autopilot has lost its clear connection to your body's center of gravity. As a result, your Autopilot has to work to keep you in what it perceives to be a balanced position, even though you are at rest. This is very common. However, when your body is at rest, you shouldn't have to be working at all. That's why we call it rest.

Most people find that they feel off-center when they do this Autopilot Assess for the first time. If you're not sure what you feel, that means you're having a hard time using just your Body Sense to sense what you feel. And if you're having trouble when you're thinking about it, imagine how hard your Autopilot is working when you are not.

To better understand how your Body Sense and Autopilot work, I want you to try two more self-assessments. Read the instructions first and then do the assessments.

Body Scan Assess

▶ *Stand with your feet side by side and close your eyes.*

▶ *Scan up your legs using your Body Sense. Are your thigh muscles engaged? Are you squeezing your butt cheeks? See if you can release these muscles and still remain upright.*

If you sensed that your butt and thigh muscles were engaged, your Autopilot is operating inefficiently, which is causing your body to work too hard during simple tasks. These muscles are meant for movement, not for standing. If these muscles have to contract to keep you stable when you are still, imagine how hard they have to work when you move.

Here's another standing assessment, the Autopilot Assess. Again, read the instructions and then do the assessment.

Autopilot Assess

▶ *Still standing with your eyes closed, lift all ten toes off the ground. Keep your toes lifted and take three full breaths.*

▶ *Take an inhale, and on an exhale, drop all ten toes back to the floor. Notice what you feel.*

When you dropped your toes back to the floor, did you notice your body weight drift forward? If so, you have identified that your Autopilot is unable to accurately locate your center of gravity. To compensate, the Autopilot moves your pelvis forward in order to pick up the signal of where your head, ribs, and pelvis are in relationship to your feet.

When your Body Sense is inhibited, your Autopilot has to rely more heavily on your senses of sight and touch to keep you balanced. You may have to use the arm of a chair to go from sitting to standing, look at the ground with every step you take, or hold on to a railing when you walk down a flight of stairs. This is a sign of inefficiency and can be exhausting. Ultimately, your joints can misalign, muscle contraction can become delayed, and compensation can arise, leaving you susceptible to injury.

Try the Autopilot Assess again, this time with your eyes open.

▶ **With your feet side by side, lift all ten toes off the ground and pause for a couple of breaths.**

▶ **Take an inhale, and on an exhale, drop all ten toes back to the floor. Notice what you feel.**

You may notice less of a drift, or none at all. This is because your Autopilot is using your sense of sight for assistance. When you have to rely on your vision or your Autopilot can't find your center of gravity, your movements become delayed, unstable, stiff, and labored. (And as you may have noticed, your sense of vision doesn't get better as you get older.)

Stuck stress is the cause of poor reception in the Autopilot and the loss of connection between the body's center of gravity and the joints. Stuck stress in the connective tissue and nervous systems interrupts communication between your center of gravity and the rest of your body. You don't lose your ability to remain stable and upright, but you lose the ability to do so efficiently. This depletes your energy. Over time, you can end up with neck and low back compression and misaligned joints. Symptoms such as joint pain, exhaustion, and anxiety are often the result. You may feel uncoordinated or even end up injured.

When the Autopilot regulates stability in a perpetual state of compensation or stress, it begins to affect all the other systems of the body. So what starts out as a sense of stiffness, joint ache, and postural misalignment begins to cause seemingly unrelated issues, such as midday fatigue, slow metabolism, irritability, constant hunger, and lack of focus. What's worse is, as exhausted as you may be in the middle of the day, when you try to fall asleep, you can't or you have difficulty staying asleep. This causes even more problems because sleep is when the Autopilot restores, repairs, and reboots your body. Without restorative sleep, you start the day with more stuck stress.

When you support your Autopilot and help it reacquire its connection to your precise center of gravity, bringing the satellites back online, efficiency of movement and function of all bodily systems improve.

No physical exercise or method of thinking can return the Autopilot to efficiency. It just doesn't work that way because it's an involuntary system. What I am going to teach you is how to access the Autopilot in a way that gives it the opportunity to reclaim its connection to your center of gravity and improve its efficiency. I am also going to teach you how to maintain that connection and heighten your Body Sense without putting added stress on the nervous system. Reconnecting with assessment techniques is an important part of the MELT Method and the doorway to the Autopilot. To understand why, I want to tell you the story of how MELT assessments were created before MELT was ever a method.

One day I was doing a bodywork session with a wonderfully inquisitive client named Lynn, who had chronic neck pain and severe TMJ (jaw pain). During my standard assessment process, I mentioned that her spine was very compressed. She asked, "How can you tell? Can you show me what you are feeling?"

I saw this as an opportunity and a challenge. Was there a way for her to feel or sense the imbalances in her body? If so, maybe she could recognize the root causes of her TMJ and chronic neck pain.

I had an idea. I asked Lynn to lie on the floor so her body would be resting on a hard surface. I wanted to see if she could feel the same misalignments in her posture that I had identified. Could she sense the big arch in her back? Could she feel that one shoulder was digging into the floor? Could Lynn notice that she was lopsided? I pointed out these imbalances and used my hands to help her feel what I had assessed. Lynn could feel her own misalignments, and she could identify the misaligned areas of her body that were affecting her neck and jaw. For the first time, she understood what I meant when I said that the root cause of her jaw pain was not in her jaw.

I had Lynn get back on my table again so I could do my usual hands-on treatments. When I was done, I asked her to return to the floor and see what she felt. She gasped and said, "I feel the difference. Wow!" She could feel that her shoulder blade was in a better position, her body was more balanced from side to side, and she was breathing much easier. Then she said, "Sue, what can I do on my own to make the changes last longer?"

That was the moment my obsession began. I wanted to find out if there was a way for my clients to perform techniques on themselves that could create the same kind of results that my hands-on bodywork would—without my hands. I poured all my focus, time, energy, and everything I had into this new idea. As I experimented on myself, I needed to know if anything was working. I knew how to assess my clients with my hands and eyes to identify if I had successfully rebalanced nervous system regulation, rehydrated connective tissue, or decompressed joints. There were no self-assessments for these changes that could be repeated with any accuracy that I knew of. Most assessments focused on the musculoskeletal system. Others required the use of a mirror or photographs, which meant my perception could skew the result or my body position could change when I reassessed. I had no idea how to assess repeatedly to determine whether anything therapeutic was occurring to me.

After trying to modify many fitness assessments and physical and manual therapy diagnostics, I returned to the assessment I had unknowingly created with Lynn. I learned that I could easily and accurately assess my alignment by lying on the floor. What my body felt like on the floor gave me a static baseline from which I could make an accurate comparison. It was a lightbulb moment. I sensed my body in relationship to the floor using the reference point of anatomical zero. This is the reference point for ideal joint alignment in a human body and the foundation of all anatomical models.

No human being is ever in perfect anatomical alignment. Ideal alignment is just that—an idea of what ideal is. However, the more your posture is in chronic misalignment, the more pain and chronic issues you will experience. By evaluating improvements in my alignment in a completely relaxed position, I could know if I was making changes in the systems that are responsible for joint alignment, the connective tissue and nervous systems.

Lying on the floor became my benchmark assessment. I would lie on the floor, assess my alignment, manipulate my body in different ways with various tools, and lie on the floor again to see if I felt changes. It worked! I was making the same types of changes that gave my clients relief and improved their health and function—on myself. In addition to improvements in my alignment, I noticed I felt better overall. I had great energy, even after a full day of seeing clients. I was sleeping better, and I needed less recovery after working out. I felt younger, and people were commenting on how great I looked on a daily basis.

I was beyond amazed—I was stunned. I couldn't believe that I might have created something that had the potential to help people help themselves in a completely new way. I was as much in awe of my body's healing capacity as I was unsure as to how the changes were occurring. How would I explain it to people? What would they say? Even though I was filled with questions and self-doubt, I knew I couldn't keep this to myself. I cautiously showed Lynn and a few other clients some of the basic techniques I had come up with to see if it worked on them. I wanted to see if they could sense what had shifted in their bodies, so I had them do the self-assessments too.

This presented me with a whole new set of challenges. I had spent years studying anatomy and had learned even more by having my hands on hundreds of clients. I could effortlessly use my knowledge of the human body to compare what I felt when lying on the floor before and after self-treatment. Now I had to articulate this.

I tried to teach my clients anatomy so they could assess their own posture with anatomical landmarks. This did not go so well. Asking people to value their pelvic placement and thoracic spine, or assess their cervical curve, was a lot! Their eyes glazed over, and the assessment was taking over half of our appointment time. I asked myself: How could I describe ideal alignment if my clients didn't have an understanding of anatomical landmarks? How could I make the assessment simple and consistent?

I decided to take a whole-body approach. I noticed when I would lie on the floor that my body felt like waves, alternating between areas that were heavy and light. Instead of describing anatomy, I started describing the areas of the body that should be weighted to the floor as "masses" and those that should be off the floor as "spaces." I could simply describe ideal alignment using the "masses and spaces" model so my clients could compare what they felt in relationship to what I described.

It took me years to refine the simple self-assessment that I now call the Rest Assess. This is when the language of MELT began to emerge. During this process, new discoveries about the Rest Assess came to light. I started compiling data on what misalignments my clients felt, and I found there were common imbalances. I started describing these imbalances as part of the Rest Assess as an additional comparison in contrast to ideal alignment. I realized that by sensing the symmetry of the right and left half of my body, I could also evaluate whether my Autopilot could sense my body's true center of gravity. This may sound simple, but it was an extraordinary discovery. Evaluating the masses and spaces and the Autopilot without the use of my hands or eyes became central to self-assessment. The process needed was more internal and yet more objective at the same time. I started teaching people to use only their internal awareness, or Body Sense, to assess themselves.

When I started teaching MELT to groups, I began to realize how compelling the Rest Assess truly was. At the end of class, I would look across the room at the dozens of people lying on the floor and see remarkable changes in alignment and body ease.

I could hardly believe what I was seeing. More incredibly, I was hearing from them that they sensed—and could articulate—these changes. What I was witnessing was beyond my imagination. It's difficult to describe the feelings of amazement, joy, excitement, and elation I felt when I first saw this. To my surprise, I still get the same charge at the end of every class. What is more exciting is that I can help people make changes on their own—without ever touching them!

Now it's your turn to do the full Rest Assess and evaluate your body for stuck stress.

There are three areas stuck stress loves to live: the shoulder girdle, the diaphragm, and the pelvis. Using Body Sense, instead of using vision, you'll learn what it feels like to have stuck stress in your body one area at a time.

When you assess each area, lie on your back with your palms face up, arms and legs extended. Take a few breaths and, with your eyes open or closed, begin to sense your body.

Sensing Stuck Stress in the Upper Body

Stuck stress in the upper body, or shoulder girdle, directly alters the position of the head, arms, and ribs.

Without moving, sense your head, arms, and torso. Using Body Sense, notice if you feel your head is tilting back or resting off center, if one arm feels more weighted than the other, or if you are sensing all of your upper back weight on your shoulder blades rather than feeling the mid-back (where women define the bra line) weighted to the floor. If you sense one or more of these imbalances, you have identified stuck stress in your upper body, specifically your shoulder girdle.

Let's try a movement assessment: Gently turn your head right and left. If you feel that you can turn your head farther to one side than the other, or you feel tension or pain at any point, or your shoulders move or lift as you turn your head, you have identified stuck stress in the shoulder region.

Sensing Stuck Stress in the Diaphragm

Stuck stress in the diaphragm directly alters the size and shape of the low back curve.

Notice your low back space. Ideally, the curve of the low back is a small distinctive space below the belly button. Don't touch your low back, but if you need to, put your finger in your belly button and notice whether the curve of your low back ends above that point.

If the curve feels significantly higher than the belly button, that's a sign of stuck stress in the diaphragm.

Pause and take a breath. Does your breath feel limited or restricted? If so, this is another sign of stuck stress in your diaphragm.

Sensing Stuck Stress in the Pelvis

Stuck stress in the pelvis directly alters the position of the pelvis and legs.

Bring your attention to your lower body. There are several signs of stuck stress in the pelvis: Notice if your tailbone feels like it is resting on the floor more than your butt cheeks (or if one buttock feels more weighted than the other). Another common sign of stuck stress is if one or both thighs aren't weighted on the floor. Notice if your knees are touching the floor, if the calves feel light or offset, or the feet feel like they are pointed anywhere besides northeast/northwest (like a letter *V*). All of these are signs of stuck stress in the pelvis.

Assess Your Autopilot

Divide your body into left and right sides and sense if either side of your body feels more weighted or one leg feels longer. If you are sensing this uneven feeling, you have identified Autopilot Inefficiency.

▶ Masses and Spaces

To better understand what you just assessed, think of your body as a series of masses and spaces. The relationship between the two is what creates ideal alignment. The primary masses of the body are the head, rib cage, and pelvis. The primary spaces of the body are the neck and the belly/low back curve. (Although there are vital spaces between each rib, I define the rib cage area as a mass.) In your arms and legs, the bones—your thighs and upper arms, for instance—are considered masses, and the joints—like the knees and wrists—are the spaces. Repetition and aging can cause you to lose space between the masses of your body, which creates compression and misalignment. This puts strain on your joints and can cause pain and inflammation.

When your movements or postures cause any two masses to get too close together, the space between them is compressed while another space in the body's architecture increases. This happens all the time—when you side bend at your waist, your ribs get closer to your pelvis on one side and farther apart on the other. The Autopilot regulates this balancing act to protect the organs and keep you upright, balancing and stabilizing each mass over each space in the most efficient way available.

Repetitive movements and postures lead to chronic compression of the spaces and misalignment of the masses. When you carry a heavy bag over one shoulder, lean on one leg, or hold your body in a certain position to reduce pain, the spaces compress so the masses can shift to allow your body to remain upright. Over time these temporary compensations become a fixed part of how your Autopilot regulates your whole body balance and alignment. Compensation is at best a temporary fix, however. Over time your neck and low back curves adapt to your repetition, and ultimately, pain arises due to compression in the disks of your spine and other joints.

Think about how your body adapts to sitting at a computer. The pelvis tucks under, the ribs round back, the shoulders round forward, and the head tilts forward. For hours at a time, your Autopilot has to support this posture. Then you stand up. You're no longer sitting at your desk but your pelvis is still tucked, your back is hunched over, and your shoulders are rounded. When you walk through a door, your head enters before your body does.

Every time you MELT, you'll use the Rest Assess to sense how the masses and spaces rest. The masses and spaces are also used as reference points in all the techniques to identify the proper body position and placement.

❱ Ideal Alignment and the Autopilot

Human science defines ideal alignment as "the point where all the joints align at their centers." If they are aligned, they can move in their full range of motion with minimal compression and compensation. Your Autopilot is always creating what it perceives as the most efficient alignment possible. But over time your repetitive movements and postures cause your Autopilot to perceive a less-than-ideal alignment as being normal.

The Rest Assess provides the opportunity to "check in" and evaluate your current body position in relationship to ideal alignment using the masses and spaces. The Rest Assess lets you Reconnect with where your body is imbalanced or not ideally aligned. Your body wants to be balanced and efficient. This desire is innate within all of us. When you use your Body Sense to identify that you have misalignments and imbalances, your Autopilot pauses and gets a message to tune in, connect, and take a look around. Your Autopilot resets its connection to your GPS and does a sweep of the whole body and all of its systems. The Rebalance, Rehydrate, and Release techniques can then help you return to better alignment and regulation.

The Rest Assess also gives you the opportunity to identify and address subtle pre-pain signals so you can proactively return your body to balance before pain and other symptoms arise. The ability to tap into and restore the Autopilot's regulation of your alignment is a new discovery that has been missing from therapeutic interventions.

❱ Common Imbalances

Although ideal alignment is a useful reference point, no living person is in ideal alignment. The repetitive motions of life are dehydrating and that causes stuck stress, which creates imbalances in the body.

As I worked with thousands of people, I found that there were imbalances that many, if not most, people had. These common imbalances also became a valuable reference point as they gave me a way to help people realize what they were feeling, so they could sense their own stuck stress.

These common imbalances occur in the three regions of the body where stuck stress is most prevalent—the shoulder girdle, the diaphragm, and the pelvis. I refer to these areas as the places stuck stress loves to live.

In this chart, you will see what it would feel like if there were no stuck stress in these regions, as well as the imbalances you might feel if you have stuck stress living there.

	Ideal Alignment	Common Imbalances
Stuck stress in the shoulder girdle	Your head rests at its center, behind the bridge of your nose. Your arms are evenly weighted to the floor. The heaviest part of the torso is the mid-rib wall (bra line). Your head turns easily from left to right.	Your head feels tilted back or off-center. Your arms are unevenly weighted. Your torso feels weighted on the shoulder girdle or upper third of the back. You sense limited range or pain as you turn your head from left to right.
Stuck stress in the diaphragm	You sense a small, distinct space between the navel and pelvis.	You sense a mid-back arch, above the navel, or you feel no curve at all in the low back.
Stuck stress in the pelvis	It feels like you're resting on two butt cheeks, evenly weighted from side to side. The backs of your thighs feel evenly weighted on the ground. Your knees feel evenly off the ground. Your calves feel evenly on the ground. Your ankles feel off the ground. Your heels are on the ground with your toes pointed like a letter *V* toward where the ceiling meets the walls.	You sense that your tailbone is weighted to the floor more than your butt cheeks, or your butt cheeks feel unevenly weighted. The backs of your thighs feel off the ground on one or both sides. The backs of the knees feel like they're on the floor. Your calves feel unevenly weighted or off the floor. Your ankles feel on the ground. Your feet point toward the sides of the room or straight up.

As I continued to work with people, I began to realize there are four of these imbalances that almost everyone had. Every client who had pain had at least two of these, and they could sense them—without my touching them at all. Even people who said they didn't have chronic pain also had these four common imbalances.

- Sensing all your upper back weight resting on the shoulder girdle or upper third of the back

- Sensing an extreme mid-back arch instead of a distinct low back curve

- Sensing your tailbone on the floor rather than evenly weighted butt cheeks

- Sensing that the backs of your thighs are off the ground

If left unaddressed, these imbalances cause compression and misalignment in the spine that can turn into chronic pain and other issues. By identifying these imbalances, you can begin eliminating them so they don't accumulate and cause pain over time.

Try the Rest Assess again, only this time, scan your body for the four most common imbalances and see how many of these specific things you feel.

Rest Assess

▶ *Lie on the floor, with your arms and legs straight and relaxed, palms face up. Take a breath and allow your body to relax into the floor.*

▶ *Assess stuck stress in your shoulder girdle. Does your upper body feel heaviest on your shoulder girdle rather than the middle of your rib cage?*

▶ *Assess stuck stress in your diaphragm. Does your low back curve feel more like a mid-back curve?*

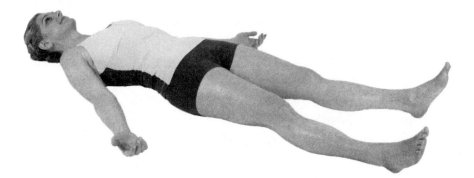

▶ *Assess stuck stress in your pelvis. Does your pelvis feel more weighted on the tailbone rather than the butt cheeks? Do the backs of your thighs feel unevenly weighted or entirely off the floor?*

▶ *If you noticed any of those four things, you have begun to learn what it feels like when there is stuck stress in your body.*

▶ Before and After

The path to pain-free, balanced health begins with Reconnect because it's what makes the other three R's of MELT work as well as they do. To create lasting changes in your Autopilot and treat the effects of stuck stress—connective tissue dehydration, compression, NeuroCore imbalance, and faulty Body Sense—you have to assess and reassess your body. This is the MELT protocol: Reconnect before and after the other three R's. Remember, to know which MELT moves to perform, you will follow a MELT map—a series of sequences combined in a particular order to achieve a desired result. A MELT map always includes all Four R's of MELT. In the following chapters, I will teach you more techniques that correspond with specific MELT moves.

In any MELT map, you will Reconnect before and after each sequence. Initially, this is how you'll know you are doing it right. You can inventory the changes you are making and track your progress. Any positive changes you experience are a sign that your connective tissue and nervous systems are responding, stuck stress is releasing, and your regulators are rebalancing. However, assessment is more than a before-and-after comparison. When you reassess and consciously connect with the changes you've made, your Autopilot resets to a more efficient, balanced state and its connection with your center of gravity is more precise and integrated. Your nervous system is de-stressed and your mind-body communication and connection is heightened. It's as if you have actively stepped in and allowed your Autopilot to recalibrate. Another profound result occurs: your restore regulator gets the opportunity to be dominant while you are awake—an extraordinary benefit to your short- and long-term health.

You don't need a tape measure, mirror, or anything except your Body Sense and the simple MELT assessments. You will use your Body Sense, or internal awareness, to assess your body's current state and whether you have the common signs of the four effects of stuck stress. Your Autopilot can't keep you balanced and stable without good Body Sense. By consciously using your Body Sense as your assessment tool, you improve its function when you're not thinking about it at all. This is an important part of getting out and staying out of pain—and keeping your body healthy. With each Assessment, you will learn your unique anatomical landscape, identify what needs your attention, connect to your regulation system, track your progress, and heighten your mind-body connection.

Remember, all systems of the body are connected, supported, monitored, and regulated by the Autopilot. Connecting to your Autopilot activates the healing mechanisms of your body while you're awake. Make sure to always Reconnect as part of your MELT self-care routine. If you don't, you will miss the opportunity to restore the link between the autonomic nervous system and the connective tissue system and address the root cause of the four effects of stuck stress.

Assessing is also your tool to catch the pre-pain and pre-symptom signals. You no longer need to be passive and simply respond to what is happening to your body. You no longer need to wait for pain as the signal that it's time to take action. Instead, you can proactively care for yourself and your body, making positive changes before pain ever starts. This is an important part of becoming a Hands-Off Bodyworker: learning self-assessment and knowing how to make lasting changes to your body with the Four R's.

I believe that self-assessment using Body Sense must be part of the protocol for any neurofascial treatment. For now, to my knowledge, MELT offers the only Autopilot self-assessment techniques.

Why We Reconnect Before and After

My discovery about the importance of Reconnecting before and after each sequence happened several years after that first assessment in my office with Lynn. Someone to whom I taught the MELT techniques came to me and said, "I think once you do MELT for a while, it doesn't really work as well or last as long."

I asked him, "What do you mean it's not working? When you assess, don't you feel the changes?"

He replied, "Well, I already know what the benefits are, so I don't really assess anymore."

I didn't really anticipate what would come out of my mouth next. "Well, how do you know if it's working if you don't assess and then value the changes? It's not about you knowing or feeling the changes; it's about your autonomic nervous system recognizing the changes. You want to connect with your nonthinking self to communicate your attempt to support it. If you don't pause and let your Autopilot sense your body's imbalances, how will your body know you are doing anything for it at all?"

I realized that I had never articulated this before. It made perfect sense to me. If you don't Reconnect before and after each sequence, you miss out on more than half of the results of MELT because your Autopilot doesn't recognize that you are imbalanced and out of alignment, so it doesn't get a chance to recalibrate. That's when I realized that the assessment was actually a powerful part of MELT self-treatment. Assessment before, during, and after each MELT sequence is necessary to create the most lasting changes in the body. Reassessing gives the Autopilot the opportunity to reacquire its GPS signal. That is why I call the first of the Four MELT R's Reconnect.

It's said that the mind can learn great things about the body through self-awareness. What I have found is that by pausing and becoming self-aware about the current state of the body, you can change how the body communicates with the mind.

▶ Reconnect to Your Center of Gravity

Reconnect is more than just assessment. Reconnect techniques also help the Autopilot reacquire and heighten its connection to your center of gravity.

To better understand the importance of this connection, I want you to try a Reconnect move called Gentle Rocking. Remember, your Autopilot is constantly working to keep your body in balance. This move helps your Autopilot reconnect to your center of gravity by challenging your balance on the unstable surface of the roller.

The techniques of MELT require a MELT Soft Roller, which can be purchased at www .meltmethod.com, along with the Hand and Foot Treatment Kit and the companion DVDs. If you don't have a soft roller yet, you can try these techniques by using rolled-up beach towels or a traditional, firm roller wrapped in a towel, blanket, or yoga mat.

First, get on the roller.

▶ *Sit next to the bottom of the roller and lean away from it. Put your hands behind you, and then shift your pelvis onto the roller.*

▶ *Using your hands for support, slowly roll yourself down along the length of the roller.*

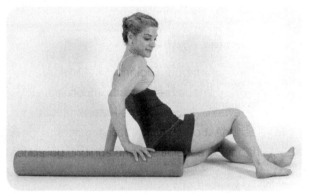

▶ *Touch the top of your head to make sure it is fully supported by the roller. Make sure your pelvis is on the roller and your feet are flat on the floor, approximately hip-width apart.*

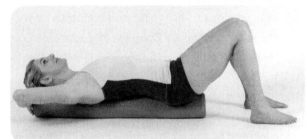

▶ *Place your forearms on the floor and take a breath.*

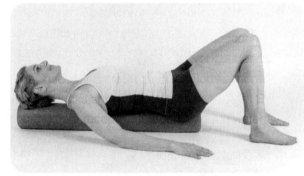

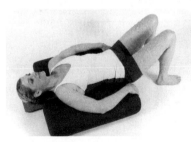

If you need additional support, place towels, pillows, or bolsters on either side of the roller.

Gentle Rocking

▶ *Allow your head, chest, and pelvis to slowly tip toward the floor on one side. Then come back through the center and slowly tip toward the other side. You want to get a sense of gently falling and catching yourself with your forearm, while keeping the*

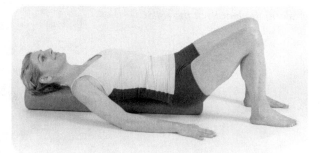

back of your head, your spine, and the center of your pelvis aligned and heavy on the roller at all times. Continue to gently rock from side to side for about 30 seconds. This move is small and subtle when done correctly.

▶ *Return to the center.*

▶ *Slowly come off the roller by placing your hands on the floor, straightening out one leg, and sliding off that side—first with your pelvis, then your ribs and head.*

Gentle Rocking helps the Autopilot go into action to keep you balanced on an unstable surface, which improves its connection to your center of gravity. Your Autopilot also uses Body Sense to track the weight of your body and the position of your joints as you gently rock side to side.

This move will become easier as you start to eliminate stuck stress in your body and improve whole-body communication by doing this and other MELT moves and sequences. Best of all, your body's ability to remain stable and balanced during day-to-day activities will improve as you support your Autopilot.

The Reconnect techniques are subtle but powerful. I discovered a doorway into the deepest aspects of the nervous system and the link between the autonomic nervous system and the connective tissue system. You now have the ability to rebalance the regulators of your autonomic nervous system to help improve your alignment, reduce pain, support the regulation of your organs, and heighten the healing state of your body. The aspects of your body's regulation that are considered involuntary are now within your reach. This type of treatment was previously possible only through a third party, such as a hands-on therapist. Now this self-care treatment is in your own hands.

6

Rebalance

There are literally thousands of books promising to help you flatten your abs, improve your core stability, and rid yourself of back pain if only you will strengthen your abs. But "core exercises" may not help you. Ironically, the very abdominal exercises many of us do to create a flat stomach and a stable spine could actually inhibit core stability and increase your chances of having a paunch.

Core and spinal stability and whole body balance are all regulated by the Autopilot. I think you'll be amazed at how much is occurring to keep you upright and stable without your conscious awareness. Reflexes are involuntary responses to changes in your body's position or the ground underneath. Even as you are sitting and reading this book, there is a whole body orchestration of reflexes so you can turn the page or touch your screen with your hand while the rest of your body stays still.

▶ NeuroCore Stability

I have identified a physiological system that the Autopilot uses to create this involuntary, reflexive stabilization. This system has two mechanisms that include connective tissue, nerves, and muscle. Together, the Reflexive and Rooted Core mechanisms work to keep you stable and upright while protecting your spine and vital organs. Here's how they work.

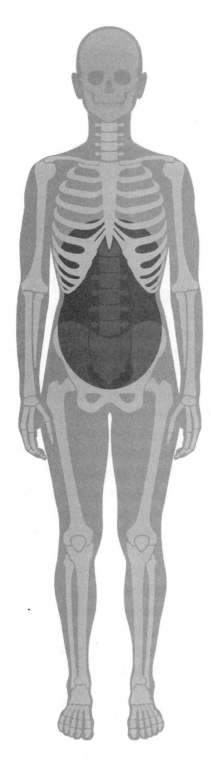

The **Reflexive Core** mechanism is an identifiable double layer of connective tissue that creates a cylinder around the organs within your torso. This egg-shaped container is strong yet pliable. Inside, a three-dimensional web of seamless connective tissue supports the organs and connects the deep stabilizing muscles. The Reflexive Core mechanism's purpose is to support and protect your vital organs and spine.

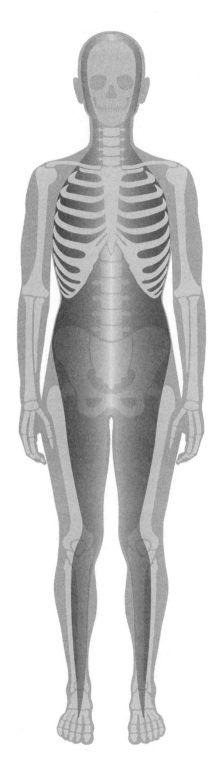

The **Rooted Core** mechanism is an identifiable channel of connective tissue, deep within your body, that runs from head to toe. This channel provides the compartments for and connection between the bones, muscles, and organs that it surrounds and intersects. The Rooted Core channel shares the same connective tissue that creates the core cylinder with the Reflexive Core. The Rooted Core mechanism grounds you and works with gravity to lift you upward and keep your masses balanced over your spaces. The purpose of the Rooted Core mechanism is to support and protect your spine while it maintains a grounded connection to the earth.

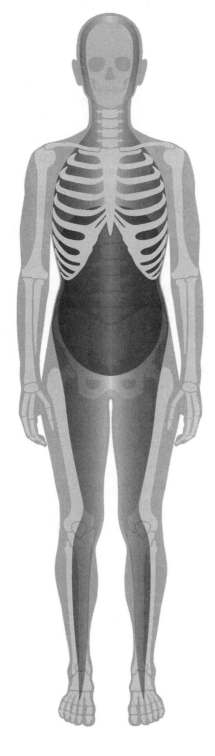

These mechanisms coordinate with dedicated, deep stabilizing muscles to do their jobs. These muscles are constantly responding to vibrational communication within the connective tissue system—not to your conscious thought. The connective tissue, nervous, and muscle system components of the Reflexive and Rooted Core mechanisms are all operating in response to an enormous amount of Body Sense information being transmitted within and between these two mechanisms. The mechanisms are always working and operate together as a system. I call this system the **NeuroCore**. The Autopilot regulates the NeuroCore system, and when it is working properly, the relationship of your masses and spaces is optimal and you are able to move effortlessly without compensation, pain, or injury. If the NeuroCore system were made up of only muscles, it would be much easier to explain. The connective tissue and nervous system components of the NeuroCore are far more complex yet important to understand in order to achieve a pain-free, healthy life.

Let's look at the Autopilot to make sense of how the NeuroCore creates upright stability. The Autopilot is constantly tracking your body position through the information it receives from the satellites, or receptors, in your joints. The Autopilot tracks your center of gravity through the vibrational communication that is being relayed within and between the Reflexive and Rooted Core mechanisms. Simultaneously, the Autopilot is tracking your primary masses—your head, ribs, and pelvis—in relation to your feet and gravity. Each of these masses contains one or more curved structures made of connective tissue.

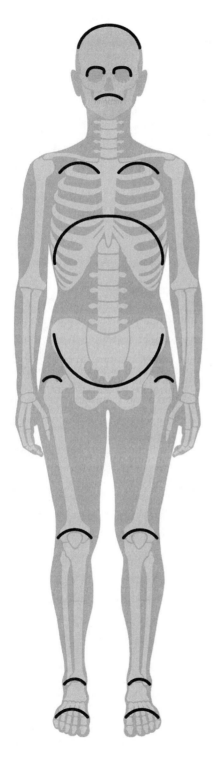

I call these structures the **domes and arches** of your body. The Reflexive and Rooted Core mechanisms rely upon seamless, vibrational communication from your feet to your head through the domes and arches. The domes and arches also play a critical role in providing buoyancy and shock absorption for the body during movement. Communication, shock absorption, and buoyancy of the domes and arches all rely on the healthy, fluid state of the connective tissue system.

The Diaphragm and Stability

While the act of breathing keeps you alive, diaphragmatic motion is essential to upright posture, dynamic movement, and vibrational communication. The diaphragm's ability to fully move is the foundation of Autopilot and NeuroCore efficiency.

The respiratory diaphragm is the primary dome in your rib cage. Think of the diaphragm as the center of communication in your body: every time you take a breath—twenty-eight thousand times a day—the movement of the diaphragm creates vibrational communication with the rest of the body and initiates numerous responses. The diaphragm and its motion creates the link between the Reflexive and Rooted Core mechanisms and helps the Autopilot sustain its connection to your center of gravity. In order to maintain an accurate signal, the diaphragm must be able to move in its three-dimensional range.

Every time you inhale, the diaphragm contracts down and out, which draws air into your lungs. Your Reflexive Core expands, and your organs gently move and glide to make room for your breath. When you exhale, your diaphragm ideally relaxes and returns to its lifted, dome-like position. At the same time, the Reflexive Core gently contracts, supporting the spine, belly, and organs. This motion stimulates the Rooted Core mechanism—the other half of the NeuroCore—to acquire a head-to-toe grounding signal by sending vibrational information to the other domes and arches of the body. Stuck stress in the diaphragm can inhibit this natural, reflexive process. The 3-D Breath Breakdown and 3-D Breath allow you to access the diaphragm and influence its movement to rebalance the NeuroCore.

Muscles and Stability

To understand the muscle system's role in creating stability, you need to know that there are two categories of muscle contraction. One type is a voluntary contraction that creates movement. The other type is an involuntary muscle contraction that stabilizes your joints and spine and protects your organs whether you're sitting, running, or at rest. I call the muscles that do these two types of jobs movers and stabilizers.

The muscles found in the mechanisms of the NeuroCore are the most essential stabilizers of your body and operate outside of your conscious control. The NeuroCore is signaled by the Autopilot, not the brain. When the NeuroCore and the Autopilot are free of stuck stress and functioning efficiently, stabilization is efficient. However, when the stabilizing mechanisms are inefficient, the muscles that usually move you are called upon to aid in stabilization. This makes movement more difficult and taxing. If muscle movers are contracting to stabilize you, when you need these muscles to create movement they are less accurate and compensation or injury is the inevitable result.

Differentiation and Stability

To sustain the space of your joints, you must be able to move your masses without compromising the spaces. I refer to the ability to isolate movement as differentiation. When the Autopilot and NeuroCore mechanisms are stabilizing you efficiently, differentiation naturally occurs. For example, when you reach for a glass from a cabinet, ideally what you see is your arm move. If stuck stress interferes with this movement, your shoulders and ribs must elevate to allow your arm to reach, and you don't even realize it. The joints of your neck and shoulder are compressed and compromised, and over time you will feel discomfort in those areas.

Differentiated movement is acquired through the stabilizing muscles of the Neuro-Core and is dictated by the Autopilot. Differentiation is essential in maintaining proper alignment. If the Autopilot and NeuroCore are chronically inefficient, you will eventually not be able to move without great effort or joint ache. Something as simple as getting out of a chair can become an event when the necessary stability and differentiation are impaired. MELT will help you reacquire the ability to differentiate and reduce your risk of compressing your joints when you move.

▶ NeuroCore Imbalance

Stuck stress in the connective tissues of the Reflexive and Rooted Core mechanisms and the diaphragm causes interruptions in the vibrational communication and the fluid state of the NeuroCore. These interruptions cause imbalance in the NeuroCore, which impairs the Autopilot's ability to find the body's center of gravity. Over time, the interruptions cause the Reflexive and Rooted Core mechanisms to become imbalanced.

You may have heard that your emotions are the cause of back pain. This idea is directly related to NeuroCore imbalance. In this case, the stuck stress that triggers the imbalance is emotional stress. Regardless of what type of stuck stress initiated the imbalance of the NeuroCore, you must rebalance the Reflexive and Rooted Core mechanisms directly to resolve stuck stress accumulation.

I have found that, for most people, the Reflexive Core mechanism isn't functioning as it should. The Rooted Core mechanism has to work overtime to compensate, and the Autopilot sends distress signals. The demand on the Rooted Core becomes so great that it becomes dehydrated and fatigued. Stability becomes quite complicated. Your brain receives the distress signals and calls upon your muscle movers to stabilize your spine and support your organs. When your body is being stabilized by muscle movers, your brain and the central nervous system are now involved. This makes you mentally and physically exhausted—and you don't even know why it's happening.

Muscle movers are not meant to be constantly active like muscle stabilizers. Over time, compensating movers become tired, tight, and locked, which can lead to inflammation, spasm, and pain. When muscle movers compensate to stabilize you, it can be seen in your posture and movements. This is one reason why muscle imbalance and weakness are usually cited as the cause of misalignment. However, muscle imbalance is a *symptom* of postural misalignment, not the cause. Postural misalignment is caused by NeuroCore imbalance and Autopilot inefficiency.

Over time, the Autopilot perceives your body's chronic misalignment as being level and balanced, and it constantly tries to return you to that state. The connective tissue that surrounds and envelops the muscles becomes strained as it tries to sustain the tensional integrity in misalignment. The connective tissue system becomes dehydrated, joints lose space, shock absorption diminishes, and inflammation increases.

I believe NeuroCore imbalance is the number one cause of back injuries like bulging disks, hernias, and back spasms. Chronic pain and sudden chronic pain are frequently the result of imbalance in your NeuroCore. A history of dehydration and compensation has occurred before you ever feel the first twinge of pain. To avoid this, you need to step in and Rebalance the mechanisms.

Is Your NeuroCore Imbalanced?

How do you know if your NeuroCore isn't in optimal condition? If you frequently feel neck or low back strain or pain, you can assume your NeuroCore isn't working efficiently. You may not even notice what came before the pain—a head that juts forward, tucked pelvis, lower belly paunch, gut issues, and stiff or awkward movements are all signs of Reflexive and Rooted Core mechanisms that aren't communicating well.

Even someone who appears to be very muscular may have a poorly functioning NeuroCore. This is why many bodybuilders and fitness fanatics have inflexibility and joint damage in their spine and hips. They are unstable and don't even know it. This used to be me.

Many people try to strengthen their abs to fix their alignment. When you train the muscle movers of the core to achieve a flat stomach, or a six-pack, it can alter the deep, constant contraction of NeuroCore stabilization. Furthermore, exercising muscles to correct postural misalignment merely strengthens your body's ability to compensate and perpetuates your misaligned state. Strengthening your muscles is a good thing, but it doesn't improve NeuroCore stability.

People who practice breathing techniques, such as those done in yoga, Pilates, meditation, and martial arts, can also have NeuroCore imbalance. Just because you work with your breathing doesn't mean your diaphragm can create the full range of movement required for accurate NeuroCore signaling to the Autopilot.

Although exercise and deep breathing techniques are beneficial, they are not designed to improve the functioning of the diaphragm and the NeuroCore. You have to Rebalance and restore communication between the Reflexive and Rooted Core mechanisms so stability can return to being effortless.

I have discovered a way to tap in to the NeuroCore to Rebalance the Reflexive and Rooted Core mechanisms and restore the Autopilot's connection to your center of gravity. Immediately, whole-body communication and stability are improved, and your entire body de-stresses. What's exciting is that the NeuroCore Rebalance techniques are so simple and effective that anyone can do them and see immediate results. You no longer have to wait for pain to arise to identify and resolve NeuroCore imbalance.

▶ MELT Rebalance Techniques

MELT Rebalance techniques give you the tools to quiet your stress reflex and bring your body back into balance. The Rebalance moves shown in the following MELT sequence expand the diaphragm's three-dimensional range of movement and Rebalance the

NeuroCore system. This sequence improves balance, gut support, and spinal stability, which are an essential part of preventing or reducing any type of body pain and maintaining optimal organ function. If you are currently under a doctor's care or have any concerns about trying this or any other sequence, please consult your doctor.

Rebalance Sequence

This sequence is most effective when done in a quiet area so you are able to focus inward.

Rest Assess	**3-D Breath**
Gentle Rocking	**Rest Reassess**
3-D Breath Breakdown	

Rest Assess

▶ *Lie on the floor, with your arms and legs straight and relaxed, palms face up.*

Take a focused breath and allow your body to relax into the floor. Close your eyes and take a moment to sense what you feel. Don't adjust or touch your body—just take notice.

Remember, there are three areas stuck stress loves to live: the shoulder girdle, the diaphragm, and the pelvis. Using Body Sense, scan your body and notice what you feel.

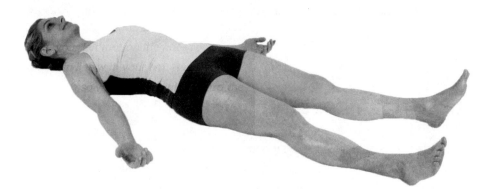

- *Assess stuck stress in your shoulder girdle. Does your upper body feel heaviest on your shoulder girdle rather than the middle of your rib cage? Is your head tilting back or resting off center? Do your arms feel out of balance?*

- *Turn your head left and right. Do you feel pain or limited range?*

- *Assess stuck stress in your diaphragm. Does your low back curve feel more like a mid-back curve?*

- *Take a focused breath. Do you sense any restriction as you inhale?*

- *Assess stuck stress in your pelvis. Does your pelvis feel more weighted on the tailbone than on your butt cheeks? Do the backs of your thighs feel unevenly weighted or entirely off the floor? Do your feet point out toward the sides of the room or up to the ceiling?*

- *Assess your Autopilot. Imagine dividing yourself into right and left sides. Does one entire side of your body feel more weighted to the floor, or does one leg feel longer than the other?*

This Rest Assess is a powerful tool that you will use throughout the book. Remember how to do the Rest Assess and come back to this section when you need to practice this technique again.

Gentle Rocking

▶ *Sit next to the bottom of the roller and lean away from it. Put your hands behind you, and then shift your pelvis onto the roller.*

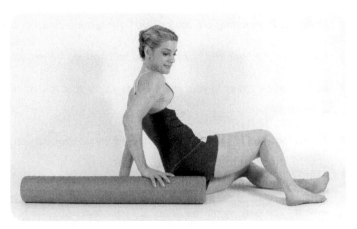

▶ *Using your hands for support, slowly roll yourself down along the length of the roller.*

If you need additional support, place towels, pillows, or bolsters on either side of the roller.

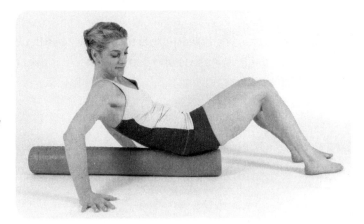

- *Touch the top of your head to make sure it is fully supported by the roller. Make sure your pelvis is on the roller and your feet are flat on the floor, approximately hip-width apart.*

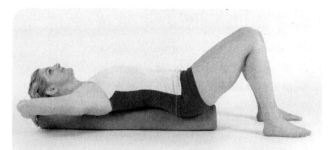

- *Place your forearms on the floor and take a breath.*

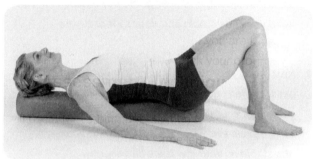

- *Allow your head, chest, and pelvis to slowly tip toward the floor on one side. Then come back through the center and slowly tip toward the other side. You want to get a sense of gently falling and catching yourself with your forearm, while keeping*

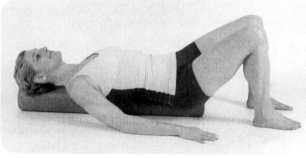

the back of your head, your spine, and the center of your pelvis aligned and heavy on the roller at all times. Continue to gently rock from side to side for about 30 seconds.

- *Every time you get on the roller, you'll start by gently rocking your body from side to side.*

- *Notice what you feel: Do you shift your body weight more easily to one side than to the other?*

- *Return to the center.*

Pelvic Tuck and Tilt

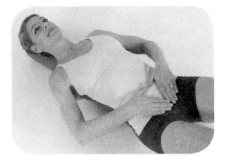

▶ *Place your hands on your pelvis, with your fingertips on the pubic bone and the heels of your hands on the front hip bones.*

▶ *Take a focused breath and slowly tuck your pelvis. When you tuck your pelvis, the heels of your hands get heavy, your low back travels toward the roller, and your pubic bone rises. Keep your ribs stable and your foot pressure constant.*

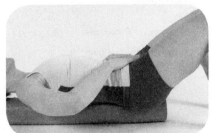

▶ *Next, keep your ribs heavy and slowly tilt your pelvis. When you tilt your pelvis, your fingertips get heavy, your pubic bone sinks, and your low back travels away from the roller. Keep your ribs stable as your low back lifts slightly.*

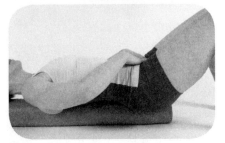

▶ *Repeat the tuck and tilt 5–6 times, moving slowly. Keep your feet light on the floor and your ribs relaxed and still.*

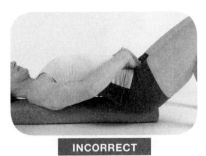

INCORRECT

Make sure you aren't squeezing your butt cheeks or lifting your hips as you tuck and tilt. Don't push into your feet to tuck or let your ribs lift away from the roller when you tilt. The size of the movement is very small and isolated when you perform this move correctly.

Remember, if you notice that your body is rocking slightly left and right, let it happen: This is a good indication that your Autopilot is reconnecting to your center of gravity.

3-D Breath Breakdown

▶ *Place one hand on your chest and the other on your belly.*

▶ *Take 3-4 breaths into the area between the front and the back of your body, allowing the diaphragm to expand from your center in two directions—front and back—as you inhale. These breaths don't need to be the fullest breaths you can take. Instead, focus on expanding your diaphragm in only two directions.*

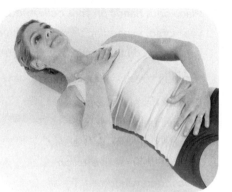

▶ *Place your hands on the widest part of your rib cage, below your armpits. Take 3-4 breaths, allowing the diaphragm to expand between your hands. Find the width of your breath. See if you can sense your hands and ribs moving apart on the inhale. The movement is subtle.*

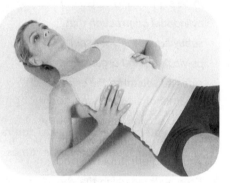

▶ *Place one hand on your collarbones, at the base of the throat, and the other on your pubic bone, at the base of the belly. Take 3-4 focused breaths between them, sending your breath all the way down to your pelvis and all the way up to the top of your lungs at the same time.*

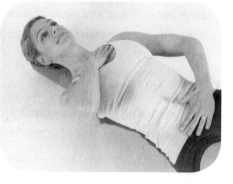

▶ *Notice if your body shifts or the roller rocks a little during any of these directional breaths. This is a good indication that your Autopilot is resetting and acquiring its GPS signal to your center of gravity.*

3-D Breath

▶ *Place both hands on your belly and take a focused breath into all six sides of your torso, expanding three-dimensionally. Notice how your belly expands into your hands on the inhale, and away from them naturally on your exhale. Try this 2–3 times.*

On your next exhale, make a firm shhh, seee, or haaa sound to heighten your ability to sense the reflexive action in your deep abdomen. Try all three sounds and sense the cylindrical contraction that subtly squeezes your spine, pelvic floor, and organs from all sides as you force the exhale.

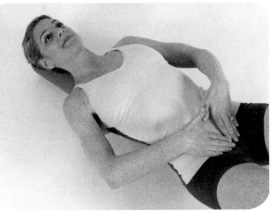

▶ *Pick the sound that best allows you to sense this inward contraction or hugging sensation in your belly, and use that sound a few more times.*

▶ *Then, without using the sound or forcing an exhale, see if you can use your Body Sense to feel and follow that same reflexive action, starting with your natural exhale and then consciously connecting to the more subtle sensation of engagement.*

▶ *Try this 2–3 times.*

▶ *Slowly come off the roller by placing your hands on the floor, straightening out one leg, and sliding off that side—first with your pelvis and then your ribs and head.*

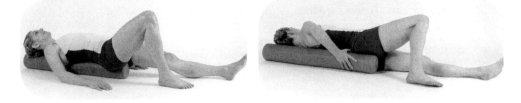

Rest Reassess

▶ *Lie on the floor with your arms and legs straight and relaxed, palms face up, as you did before. Breathe and allow your body to relax into the floor. Close your eyes and take a moment to reassess.*

▶ *Remember how your body felt when you did your Rest Assess. Use your Body Sense to notice if you've helped eliminate any accumulated stress.*

▶ *Turn your head from left to right. Do you have more range of motion? Is there less pain or stiffness as you turn your head?*

▶ *If you felt like your upper body was heaviest on your shoulder girdle, do you feel more weight in the middle of your rib cage?*

▶ *Do you feel like your low back curve is closer to your pelvis?*

▶ *If you felt like your pelvis was more weighted on the tailbone than on your butt cheeks, notice if you've made any changes there. And what about your thighs: Do they feel heavier and more evenly weighted?*

▶ *Here's the most important thing: Divide yourself into a right side and a left side. Do you feel more even and balanced from side to side? If so, you've improved your Autopilot's connection to your center of gravity, so it can function more efficiently.*

▶ *Take a breath. Do you feel like you can breathe more easily or more fully?*

▶ *If you sense any of these changes, your body is Rebalancing.*

Body Changes: After completing the Rebalance Sequence, you may notice these specific changes when you Reassess:

• Your upper body is more relaxed on the floor.

• Your breath feels fuller and more effortless.

• Your body feels more balanced from left to right.

▶ The Power of Rebalance

After you identified your imbalances, you did some rocking, some shushing, and a little focused breathing and, voilà, your body is in a new, more balanced place and your Autopilot's GPS signal is back online. Although it may seem like you didn't do much, the changes that your body made are profound.

I get excited every time I teach the Rebalance Sequence in a group environment. Watching an entire room of people transform their bodies to a balanced, settled position right before my eyes never gets old. I never take for granted the power of this simple sequence to restore essential elements of good health. It is a gift to me as much as to my students. The fact that I found a way to access the Autopilot, without my hands, is almost as mind-blowing as how I figured it out in the first place.

One morning I woke up, and I have to admit, I was hungover. I had a few too many cocktails at a friend's fortieth birthday party the night before. I felt like I had been run over by a bus. I immediately drank about a liter of water and, instead of going back to bed, decided to MELT a little to see if I could make myself feel better.

When I did the Rest Assess, I sensed that my entire body was weighted to one side. It felt as if the floor was slanted, but it wasn't. I tried to readjust myself, but the feeling remained. It felt very unusual. I had never felt so entirely out of balance during a Rest Assess.

It didn't seem like a good idea to do the MELT Rehydrate techniques—I was nauseated and my head was throbbing. So instead, I decided to try some standard diaphragmatic release techniques while lying with my spine on the roller.

After breathing into each direction of my torso, it occurred to me to then breathe into all three dimensions with a new intention. As I exhaled, I followed the natural deep contraction in my abdomen with the idea that it might help with the nausea. I focused my intent on the subtle, three-dimensional gathering that was occurring in the deep layers of my abdomen. It felt like a gentle, internal hugging sensation. My focus was not on the muscle contraction. I was focused on contacting the deepest layers of my core each time I exhaled. I knew from my manual therapy work that this contraction occurred involuntarily with every exhalation and could be improved with a variety of hands-on techniques. A wave of calm began to spread throughout my body. My head started to clear, my breathing opened up, my nausea subsided, and my jaw relaxed. It was a little miracle.

I came off the roller and reassessed. The masses of my body were much more settled into the floor. But what surprised me was that the feeling that I was leaning to one side was now totally gone. My postural alignment had radically changed just by lying on the roller and consciously connecting to what I now call the NeuroCore.

I couldn't believe it. I felt remarkably better, and the feeling lasted for the rest of the day. I didn't have to take any aspirin. I ate a good meal, drank lots of water, and even felt good enough to work out.

I wondered if this lopsided feeling was merely a by-product of my hangover or if this was something that my students would notice if they did this assessment. And if they experienced the same uneven feeling, could the instant improvement be repeated?

The next morning, after I did the usual Rest Assess at the beginning of class, I asked my students whether they sensed that one entire side of their body was more weighted to the floor or that one leg felt longer than the other. To my surprise, more than half the students in the room raised their hands.

I had everyone lie on the roller and do a 3-D Breath Breakdown followed by a full 3-D Breath. I had my students make a *shhh* sound to help them sense the subtle, involuntary contraction. During the reassess I asked, "For those of you who felt off balance from left to right before, how many of you feel more centered now?" Every single hand went up. I was shocked and excited.

They wanted to know what we had done. I couldn't fully explain it to them. I was just beginning to make sense of it myself. I had a hypothesis: "It seems as if your nervous system can better find your center of gravity now." I could see the difference, and they could feel it. Had I accidentally discovered a therapeutic technique that could actually help people create changes in their own nervous system regulation? I realized that when you consciously connect to the involuntary contraction that supports your spine and organs, your whole-body alignment improves. Now I had to figure out *how* it improved whole-body alignment. What was allowing the nervous system to regain balance? What was making the body change so quickly in such a profound way?

These questions led me to an intense period of research and experimentation, the recounting of which could fill the pages of an entire book. The result is my model of the NeuroCore. This model offers a new understanding of how the body creates stability without our conscious control. These discoveries radically change your ability to tap into and rebalance the reflexive, stabilizing mechanisms of your body. When your body is stable, connected, and aligned, it can efficiently manage all types of stress, so that stress doesn't become stuck. When you Rebalance the NeuroCore, you also stimulate the body's innate restorative healing mechanism. I now understand that what seemed like such a simple, subtle technique when I was hungover was not simple to the body. Here's the rundown of what's occurring:

Assess your Autopilot's ability to sense your center of gravity: As you learned in the Reconnect chapter, when you are at rest, you can assess your Autopilot efficiency. If your body feels heavier on one side or if one leg feels longer than the other, your Autopilot is off-kilter and having a hard time locating your center of gravity. The identification of any off-centeredness is step one.

Lie on the roller along your spine: In this position, your brain is flooded with information about your body's position because you are gently stimulating the spine with a soft roller. In a normal day, your spine never gets this type of positive, gentle compression, even when you lie on the floor. This position opens up a powerful communication channel between your hands, feet, spine, and brain.

Simultaneously, you are lying on an unstable surface, so your Autopilot is challenged to stabilize you while your spine is being stimulated. Gentle Rocking then heightens the Autopilot's GPS signal to your center of gravity. This is the first step in rebalancing the regulators and your NeuroCore.

Differentiate your pelvis: When you isolate the movement of your pelvis from your legs and ribs, you improve your Autopilot's connection to your center of gravity. The slight shifting or rocking on the roller that occurs during this movement is an indication that your Autopilot is reacquiring its GPS signal to your center of gravity.

Do the 3-D Breath Breakdown: Experiencing diaphragmatic movement through your awareness and your hands, with your spine supported by the soft roller, enhances the diaphragm's ability to move in its full range when you're not thinking about it. This opens up the communication channels between your Reflexive and Rooted Core mechanisms, which improves the Autopilot's ability to find the center of gravity.

Do the 3-D Breath: When you inhale into all six sides, you experience the diaphragm's more expansive range of motion. The greater purpose of the 3-D Breath, though, is to enhance the involuntary contraction of your NeuroCore during your exhale. This is a reflexive contraction of both stabilizing muscles and connective tissue.

When you make specific sounds, such as a *shhh*, during your exhale, it increases pressure and vibration in the abdomen. This heightens your ability to sense the reflexive, stabilizing core contraction and the gentle hugging around the organs. Then when you exhale without sound and consciously use your Body Sense to feel and follow that same involuntary contraction, you enhance its ability to occur even when you stop thinking about it.

Reassess: Identifying the change—your body resting more evenly on the floor—allows your awareness and your Autopilot to recognize your body's true center of gravity.

All six moves collectively reset the Autopilot. When your Autopilot can find your center of gravity, a rebalancing of the stress regulators occurs. That's why people often experience that immediate *ahhhh* feeling. Your muscle, organ, nervous, and connective tissue systems experience that same type of relief.

You can't think your way into a better center of gravity or a rebalancing of your stress regulators. You have to go through the body. By using Body Sense and improving vibrational communication, you can recalibrate the balance of your NeuroCore mechanisms, thereby improving communication and ridding your body of the sensation of loss of balance. And doing so is an important step in your journey to a pain-free life.

7

Rehydrate

At the start, I was obsessed with rehydration. In particular, I wanted to teach my clients how to do it for themselves. My clients always reported feeling much better after a session, so how could I teach them to achieve that feeling without me?

I became convinced that the answer could be found in the connective tissue. In my hands-on work, renewing the fluid state of this tissue system created the most immediate, lasting changes. I decided to experiment on myself. If I could figure out how to self-treat this tissue, then I could offer my clients new solutions for staying free of pain and improving overall health. I quickly learned that using my own hands to self-treat my tissue with the same subtle, light touch I used on my clients did not yield the same result. It was just not possible to be both a transmitter and a receiver of the specialized light touch vibration needed to improve the fluid state of the connective tissue in a therapeutic way. Further, it was difficult to reach particular parts of my body, like my spine and shoulders, in order to treat them. I knew I had to use a prop.

I never dreamed that one of the props I would ultimately use would be a roller.

I had never really been a fan of the foam roller.

Hard foam rollers have been used to rub out kinks and knots in muscles for more than half a century, a technique that in more recent years has been referred to as self-myofascial release. This is a method of rolling a hard foam roller back and forth under a muscle group or area of the body. The motion is similar to ironing a shirt or vacuuming a rug, with the intention of releasing muscle tension by improving blood flow. When you hit a painful spot, you roll directly over it or maintain pressure on that spot until you basically can't stand it anymore. Then you continue on with the back-and-forth motions until you find the next spot.

I was first introduced to foam rolling in my twenties. I had gone to a physical therapy office after I hurt my knee. Before my appointment, I was lying on the floor and stretching next to an athletic guy who was rolling back and forth on his outer thigh. As he grimaced and made all sorts of grunting sounds, I asked him what he was doing.

He said, "I'm getting the knots out of my IT band to help my knee."

I immediately grabbed one of the other white, hard rollers and did what he was doing. It was really painful. "Is it supposed to hurt?"

He replied, "That's how you know it's working. The more it hurts, the more it's working!"

So I went ahead and rolled back and forth over my thighs. The next day, my thighs hurt so bad I could barely feel my knees at all. The pain in my thighs was a distraction from my knee pain, but my knees didn't feel any better. Was I missing something?

For a short time, I kept trying. Rolling on a white roller felt like I was rubbing a bruise. I often felt more sore afterward than I did before. I never saw much of a positive change in my muscle issues, performance, or knee pain. Bottom line: I was trying to get out of pain, and it hurt. I talked to other athletes who used the foam roller and found out that it was supposed to hurt. And they loved the pain. I thought, why would causing pain show you that something was working? I looked for someone to explain that logic to me. No one did. So I stopped rolling.

Years later, as I learned more about connective tissue from the scientific research-ers and my own work, I understood what I had intuitively felt when I first tried foam rolling. Inflicting pain on oneself isn't a solution for pain. Remember, regardless of the underlying causes, pain is a symptom of dehydrated connective tissue. What I have found is that your connective tissue and nervous systems don't respond positively to intense, self-inflicted pressure on tissue that isn't properly prepared or allowed time to adapt. Instead, connective tissue reacts to protect the underlying nerves, blood vessels, and even muscles from being damaged by the heavy compression. The intense compression initiates a sensory nerve signal of pain to the brain in order to alert you of potential trauma or damage, like an acute injury. This causes unnecessary stress on the nervous system.

This type of fast, intense pressure can actually irritate the connective and muscle tissues as well as the nerves and vessels. The pain signal is the nerves' attempt to protect themselves from harm. Although heavy compression and deep pressure may be beneficial in particular circumstances, in my professional opinion, these techniques are ideally administered by experienced professionals who know what they are doing. If you are going to do these types of intense pressure techniques on yourself, make sure that you first learn how from a well-trained professional and that your connective tissue is hydrated. Most importantly, understand that inflicting pain should not be the ultimate goal and that pain does not indicate benefit or proper application.

Going directly after tight muscles is also not the way to get out of pain or improve performance, and it can often cause more problems. The superficial layer of connective tissue that sits above all the muscle (or myofascial) layers must be hydrated for the muscles to receive clear neurological input. Connective tissue dehydration causes uncoordinated movement, muscle fatigue, and pain. Once the tissue is rehydrated, then stretching, massage, and other light- or medium-pressure modalities can feel good and help sustain a positive change. Remember, you don't want to do things to yourself that hurt.

One popular method of relieving muscle tension is massage. I'm a big fan of massage. It's also a great way to relax the mind and body, and improve circulation. I love that someone else does it to me. Of course, that means that it costs money. The intention of a massage is different than MELT, as massage focuses on muscle and blood circulation. If you enjoy getting massages too, MELT will help the results of your massage last longer.

❱ Finding the Right Tool

When I started to experiment with manipulating my connective tissue, I realized that I had to use a prop if I wanted to simulate my hands-on treatments. I tried everything from fitness props and physical therapy tools to toys and kitchen items in order to find something that would create an effect similar to that of my hands-on work. Oddly enough, my search led me back to the foam roller, but I had to develop a much softer roller than what was available. I found that a soft roller was ideal for creating compression on the most sensitive areas of the body. The same tool could also be used for the support and gentle stimulation of the spine. Once I determined that the soft body roller was the ideal tool, I developed every technique and position in relationship to the circumference, shape, and density of that roller.

In the early years of MELT, people would assume I was using the foam roller for self-myofascial release, and I found this frustrating. I felt like I was always trying to explain how MELT wasn't like another technique or method and that the roller was quite different. What I came to realize was that I had created a completely new use for the roller.

▶ Positive Compression

In my quest, I focused first on how I could manipulate the fluid state of my connective tissue in and around a joint for the sole purpose of increasing joint space, mobility, and proper alignment, like I did in my private practice. I was doing what manual therapy would define as direct compression techniques—directly manipulating the tissue around a specific joint. I moved slowly, in small areas, with the intention of compressing the tissue while making sure to maintain tolerable pressure. I was simulating Rolfing, deep tissue, and neuromuscular techniques without allowing the pressure to get to the point of pain.

If you think about it, pain-free compression and manipulation is most precise when you do it to yourself. Only you can sense when you are at the point of pain. Even then not everyone's Body Sense or pain gauge of what is tolerable is a match for what the body needs, although this can be learned. Remember, pain heightens the stress regulator and Autopilot's protective response, which in turn causes inflammation and more pain. As a hands-on therapist, I never intentionally inflict pain. I intuitively knew that with any technique I developed, I had to keep the notion of creating pain out of the equation.

As I continued to assess, experiment with compression, reassess, and experiment some more, I made some discoveries. The tolerable compression not only stimulated an exchange of fresh, moving fluid in the joint I was focusing on, but the exchange was also occurring in a much greater area than I was compressing. I remember it being such an odd yet good feeling the first time I sensed it when I was reassessing in the Rest Assess position. It felt like my back was more open, vibrant, lighter, and yet more grounded. This was beyond sensing improved blood flow. The fluid motion I felt was directly in the matrix of connective tissue.

Although my joints felt better and moved with greater ease initially, if all I did was the compression techniques in isolated regions, the good feeling didn't last very long. An hour or two later, the area I had compressed would have minor swelling and my joints would feel stiff. I don't know if anyone else would have noticed it visually, but I felt it. This was the opposite effect of what I wanted to achieve.

I knew what was missing. In my hands-on work, after I stimulated an exchange of fresh fluid in a joint, I would make sure that the fluid movement of the local tissue was reintegrated with the movement of the greater connective tissue system. If I did that, it yielded a greater result. It wasn't enough to just pull the fluid into the joint; the fluid needed to move through the joint and beyond. Lasting change came from integrating the new fluid from the joint area into the directional fluid movement of the entire connective tissue system. Unfortunately, I had no idea how to replicate this process without using my hands.

So I tried some reverse engineering. I completely put aside the way I did this with my hands on my clients. The highly specific, light-touch vibration just couldn't be done on myself. With a few willing clients, I started using my hands and arms as if they were a roller. I would compress the joint area and then experiment with different techniques and pressures to try to reintegrate the fluid movement. I drew from what I had learned about the superficial layer of connective tissue from cadaver dissection with Gil Hedley and other scientific research about the uniqueness of this layer of connective tissue.

I intuitively knew that to integrate the fresh fluid exchange in the deep, fibrous layers of the connective tissue and the joints with the whole body, I would need the help of the superficial layer right underneath the skin. Gil helped me better understand this layer of tissue and encouraged me to continue to work with it to induce whole-body connection and integration. One day I was working on my client Bill, and it came to me to try to create a continuous sweep of light pressure after I did the compression. I used my palm and forearm to do a light sweeping motion on the area around the knee joint. I pushed the fluid in only one direction with the intention of reintegrating the fluid from around the joint all the way to the superficial layer.

It worked! When I reassessed, I was able to sense improvement in the fluid movement of the entire connective tissue system. Bill noticed a greater range of motion, ease of movement, and greater flexibility—and it lasted. This protocol of compression followed by light, directional sweeping with the roller created a lasting change in and around the joint as well as throughout the entire connective tissue system.

I tried the same technique with the roller on myself and found similar results. Then, as always, I tried it out with other willing clients. As I experimented I found even more effective ways to explain how to get the greatest results. Today in MELT, we call the technique of lightly sweeping the roller in one direction Rinsing.

◗ My Little Secret

I wasn't only trying to recreate manual therapy techniques I had learned; I was also trying to mirror some that I had developed on my own.

In my private practice, the layer of connective tissue beneath the skin, or the superficial layer, is the first thing I assess with my hands. I can sense a fluidlike vibration that moves just beneath this layer of the connective tissue. I didn't learn this or hear about it from any of my manual therapy training or higher education. It's something I've been able to feel as long as I can remember. Once I became a hands-on therapist, I gained more experience and became even more aware of what I was sensing. One thing I discovered was that wherever the vibrational fluid in the superficial layer wasn't moving in a cohesive, directional motion, those were the areas of the body that needed the most attention. When dehydrated, this outer layer could be imagined as a pair of jeans that are two sizes too small. It's uncomfortable to walk, bend over, or sit. Everything underneath the tight jeans gets squished. It can be painful.

Regardless of my clients' primary complaints or seemingly greater issues, I found that if I addressed the superficial layer with specific, organized light touch, then my ability to address areas of dehydration or stagnation in the joints, muscles, organs, and deeper connective tissues was more effective and longer lasting.

◗ A Multilayered Approach

As I continued to see greater results from self-treating the connective tissue, I was motivated to see what other manual therapy techniques could inform the techniques I was creating. Simultaneously, more scientific research was emerging about connective tissue and why manual therapy techniques are so effective. Although intuitively I understood what I felt, it was only once the science of connective tissue started to emerge that I was able to articulate just what it was I was trying to do.

The various types of receptors in the connective tissue and their responsiveness to different degrees of pressure had been discovered. Now I knew why the different types of compression applied in various states of hydration worked. I knew that when I compressed connective tissue with my hands, it was important to approach dehydrated tissue first and give it time to adapt. If I went too deep too fast, the tissue repelled my touch and fluid exchange was not possible. This is what happens with a firm roller. So I tried to ease into the pressure with the soft roller. I got a better result if I first moved gently on the roller to explore the tissue and introduce the pressure. This also allowed the layers of tissue to slowly adapt and be more receptive to the compression. Today I call this technique Gliding.

During any hands-on tissue treatment, I always did more than one type of compression on any given area in order to create the most effective fluid exchange. With this in mind, I tried what seemed like endless variations of the amount of depth and duration when compressing different areas of the body. I developed different ways of compressing each mass of the body to get the most immediate and lasting change. Today, these compression techniques are called Shearing, and there are two types: direct and indirect.

Direct and indirect Shearing are executed differently depending on which area of the body you are Shearing. I experimented with compression on every area of my body to determine the areas that were effective and safe to Shear. I learned that it is best not to compress the spaces of the body. Only a highly skilled professional should manipulate your spaces (such as the abdomen, neck, throat, and low back) so that the nerves and organs that are exposed in these areas are not harmed or injured. I have some war stories that include bruising my kidney, overstimulating nerves in my gluteal fold (ouch!), and causing a long-lasting "stitch" in my abdomen. In MELT, you will learn techniques that effectively treat the spaces by working in the masses above and below them.

▶ The Behavior of Connective Tissue

Compelling research articles started to appear. Scientists were conducting laboratory tests to see how connective tissue reacted to tension caused by mechanical pulling of the tissue. What was remarkably different about this research was that it was focused not on the muscle system but on the connective tissue and how tensional pull affected its hydration, adaptability, and responsiveness.

The research showed that when tension was applied and the connective tissue was pulled taut, it decreased the amount of fluid in the tissue. The length of time and the rate at which the tissue was pulled determined the amount and speed at which fluid returned to the area when the tension was released. Scientific studies concluded that the longer this tissue is pulled or compressed, the more difficult it is for the cells to bring fluid back into the tissue on their own and for the collagen fibers to return to their ideal length. Without adequate fluid, what's left is dehydration—what we call stuck stress—and its many potential problems over time. Fortunately, the same property that leads to connective tissue dehydration can lead to rehydration when done for a short period of time. This manual therapy hypothesis had been around for years and finally had a scientific explanation.

❱ Compression Isn't Enough

This new research inspired me to find a way to create the positive tensional pull on myself that I had done on my clients with my hands. I wanted to be able to stimulate as many receptors and layers as possible to create the greatest hydration effect. When I do this for clients, they are lying still, so I can create the pull on the connective tissue without getting their muscles involved. In order to do this to myself, I was going to need to use my muscles. How was I going to create enough tensional pull on my connective tissue without my muscles taking over? It was tricky. I explored different positions, contortions, props, and movements. Over time I discovered how to pull the connective tissue to its end range without a muscle stretch interfering. The trick was to create two-directional pull between areas of the body by moving them in opposition. The roller gave me the leverage to make that possible.

Once I was in the right position, I had to move slowly to allow the connective tissue to adapt as it found its end range. Otherwise, the muscles I was using to create the pull became primary, and it turned into a muscle stretch. As with compression, I found that it is important to pause and wait for a few focused breaths as the fluid leaves the connective tissue. Then when I released the pull, the rehydration effect occurred. Pulling the connective tissue in two directions initiated a powerful fluid exchange and immediately improved the extensibility of the tissue.

The Two-Directional Length techniques, as we call them today, are specific for each area of the body. In the MELT maps in Chapter 13, you will learn how to lengthen the connective tissue in different areas of your body.

❱ A New Kind of Treatment

What still amazes me today is that I found I could show people how to self-treat their connective tissue system and achieve the same results as I could with my hands-on techniques. At that time, the biggest challenge was shifting people's focus from inflicting pain and stretching muscles to self-treating a system of the body that no one had ever heard of before.

The process of creating and refining each MELT technique taught me so much about the connective tissue system. The connective tissue, nervous, and muscle systems are all improved by using these techniques. I am continually in awe of the body's capacity to heal itself when you address the issue of hydration. And fascial research continues to validate my hands-on findings and the science behind the MELT Method itself.

▶ Rehydrate Your Connective Tissue

When you Rehydrate your connective tissue, you dramatically increase your capacity for healing, pain-free living, and better health. You already know step one: consistently drink enough water. But if your connective tissue system isn't absorbing it, your aching joints and inflamed tissues are going to stay dehydrated. That's the thing about connective tissue—you have to effectively stimulate it to get all the cells of your body to absorb the fluid you take in. That's what MELT does.

MELT's specialized techniques and tools improve the fluid state of the connective tissue. When connective tissue is properly hydrated, the muscles work better, the joints have the support and space they need, and the whole body finds a more ideal upright alignment that helps absorb the shocks and stresses of everyday life. Even better, all the cells of your body become more receptive to absorbing the water and nutrients you consume.

Dehydration, or stuck stress, leads to body pain, joint ache, toxicity, poor posture, wrinkles, cellulite, muscle imbalance, cellular dehydration, and loads of stress on your mind and body. Specifically stimulating areas of connective tissue that are suffering from stuck stress triggers a rehydration response—it's as if the body's attention is suddenly focused on this area and what it needs to thrive. Rejuvenating the fluid in one area improves the entire connective tissue system, which I call a global rehydration effect.

Oddly, compression and tension, which dehydrate your connective tissue during repetitive activity, can also be used to Rehydrate the tissue. MELT addresses stuck stress and connective tissue dehydration with two distinct approaches: compressive stimulation and two-directional length. Here's how it works.

The connective tissue system is a three-dimensional web with definable layers and structures. Each layer contains receptors that respond to precise mechanical pull as well as light and medium, slow and fast mechanical pressure. When the receptors are positively stimulated, the fluid-producing connective tissue cells create a rehydration effect, or fluid exchange. The result of the rehydration effect is that stuck stress and inflammation decrease and the environment of all your cells and nerves improves. Manual therapists use their hands to create mechanical pressure or pull on the tissue and achieve the rehydration effect. As a Hands-Off Bodyworker, you are going to use the MELT Rehydrate techniques, the MELT soft body roller, and your Body Sense to rehydrate your connective tissue.

The MELT Rehydrate techniques include Two-Directional Length and four types of compression—Gliding, direct and indirect Shearing, and Rinsing—to stimulate the different receptors and layers of the connective tissue. These techniques create the same rehydration effect as hands-on therapy.

For MELT length techniques, the MELT soft body roller stabilizes, elevates, and gently supports your spine, ribs, or pelvis so you can attain the proper position. For the MELT compression techniques, the soft roller provides gentle, positive compression for the part of your body that is on the roller without overstimulating or stressing the connective tissue and nervous systems.

Your Body Sense, or internal awareness, is as important as the techniques and the roller to achieve the rehydration effect. You will use your Body Sense to help you identify the specific areas of your body that need extra attention. Your Body Sense will also help you identify the amount of body weight and pressure needed to achieve the specific compression for each technique.

Too much pressure when performing any of the techniques actually decreases the rehydration effect. How will you know you are applying too much pressure? Your Body Sense will send you a message: intense discomfort or pain. Pain indicates that too much pressure is being applied to positively stimulate the different connective tissue layers and receptors. Pain also overexcites the stress regulator, whereas the goal of MELT is to do the opposite and heighten the restore regulator. No part of MELT should hurt, just as I would never intentionally apply painful pressure with my hands to one of my clients. The pressure should always be tolerable, so it's important to listen to your body and make adjustments to the amount of weight you are putting on the roller if you feel pain.

▶ MELT Compression Techniques

The easiest way to learn how to do the MELT compression techniques is by doing them. Let's start with Gliding on your calf.

Calf Glide

▶ *Place the roller under the upper half of your right calf, a few inches below your knee, and cross your left ankle over your right. With your feet and legs relaxed, let your calf sink into the roller with tolerable pressure.*

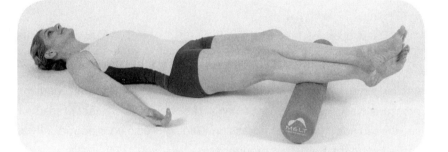

▶ *Slowly bend and straighten your knee 4–5 times to move the roller back and forth no more than 2 inches. Keep your feet and ankles relaxed, and maintain a consistent, tolerable pressure as you explore your calf for areas of stuck stress.*

▶ *Rotate your calf outward and repeat the small back-and-forth Gliding motion 3–4 times.*

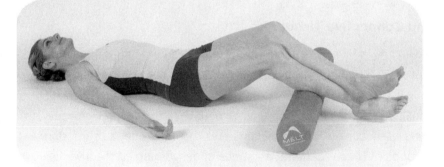

- *Then rotate your calf inward and Glide 3–4 times.*

- *Use your Body Sense to notice which of the three areas feels more tender.*

- *Return to that area and continue to Glide, making the movement smaller and smaller for 2–3 breaths.*

- *With your feet and legs relaxed, let your calf sink into the roller with tolerable pressure.*

- *Now try it on your other leg.*

Glide

In the Gliding technique, the roller is moving in small, gentle, back-and-forth movements under a small area of the body. If you compress an area of your body on the roller and the roller is moving, you are Gliding. Gliding is used to introduce a gentle exploratory pressure. Keep the movement small and slow with consistent pressure to allow the tissue time to adapt to the compression. Gliding is also your opportunity to explore the tissue to find the barriers, or tender areas, that you will then Shear.

Gliding—and all the other compression techniques—is done only on the body's masses, like the shoulder blades, hips, and thighs—never the spaces, like the neck, low back, or behind the knees. The spaces benefit from work done above and below them rather than directly on them. Your body position and roller placement for Gliding varies with which body part you are Gliding. The MELT maps in Chapter 13 include simple, step-by-step instructions for the Rehydrate techniques.

Gliding and Connective Tissue

Gliding activates the rehydration effect by introducing light to moderate compression to the part of your body that is on the roller. This lighter, softer, back-and-forth motion allows the tissue from skin to bone to adapt and prepare for the more distinct, manipulative pressure of Shearing without overstimulating the tissue. As you Glide, you will notice certain significant areas that have intense sensation, tenderness, or pain. These "barriers" are areas of dehydrated connective tissue. This is what stuck stress feels like. The discomfort is your body's signal that these areas require special attention.

The more often you MELT, the fewer barriers you will find. Note that some areas of the body, such as near the outer hip and inner thigh, especially closer to the joints, have more dense layers of connective tissue. These regions of the body are frequently strained by our repetitive postures and hold more barriers, causing muscles to become inhibited. These areas can be extremely tender, which is your cue to ease off pressure in order to achieve the most beneficial result.

Remember, you always want to maintain tolerable pressure during any of the compression techniques. Pain is your signal that the compression is too much.

Now let's try Shearing.

Calf Shear

▶ *Position your body and the roller in the same way as you did for Gliding on your right calf. Remember which of the three areas felt more sensitive when you were Gliding, and Glide to the area again to find the tender spot.*

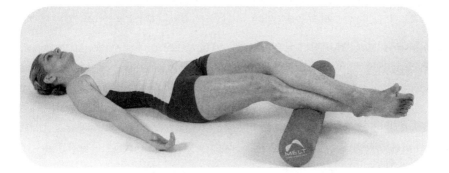

▶ *With your feet and legs relaxed, let your calf sink into the roller.*

▶ *Maintain tolerable pressure, and indirectly Shear by flexing and pointing your right ankle 3–4 times and then making circles with your ankle 3–4 times in each direction.*

▶ *Relax your ankle and create a direct Shear by turning your right leg in and out in a small, controlled movement, 1–2 inches, 4–5 times. The roller remains stationary.*

▶ *Maintain compression of your calf on the roller, and gently shift your leg slightly left to right, like you're scratching the calf against the roller. This is called cross friction.*

If you feel any pain, reduce the pressure by uncrossing your legs.

▶ *Pause, wait, and take 2 focused breaths while you let the calf sink further into the roller.*

▶ *Now try it on your other leg.*

Shear

Shearing is a more intense type of compression and stimulation and is always preceded by Gliding. There are two different ways to Shear:

Direct Shearing: The body part you are Shearing is moving on top of the stationary roller. When you rotate your leg in and out, you are directly Shearing the area of your calf. Direct Shearing stimulates the connective tissue from the outside in. Your body moves, but the roller doesn't. Instead you are creating isolated, specific movements to intensify the compression in the part of your body that is on the roller. This allows you to mobilize and rehydrate the tissue layers. The smaller the region you Shear, the better the rehydration effect.

Indirect Shearing: The body part you are Shearing stays still on the stationary roller while you move a nearby joint. You are indirectly Shearing your calf when you rotate your ankle while keeping your calf still. Indirect Shearing stimulates the connective tissue from the inside out. Moving a nearby joint while stabilizing the part of your body that is on the roller contracts and releases the muscles beneath the area you are compressing. This stimulates and hydrates the deep connective tissue layers that surround your muscles and bones.

How, when, and where you will do direct versus indirect Shearing is all outlined in the MELT maps in Chapter 13.

Shearing and Connective Tissue

Shearing stimulates the receptors found within the connective tissue to create hydration and improve the responsiveness of the tissue. Shearing effectively stimulates all the layers from your skin to your bones. It also encourages the dehydrated tissue that makes up a barrier to admit fresh fluid, allowing proper rehydration to occur. This improves the connective tissue's elastic and supportive qualities.

When you Shear, you are controlling the pressure you apply with your body weight by maintaining constant, focused pressure on the roller. The intention of this compression is to push out the fluid content (like squeezing a sponge), which stimulates the connective tissue cells to produce and take in new fluid. When you pause and wait while sustaining compression, you are pushing out all the fluid. Then when you decompress and move to the next spot, even more fluid than was there previously is pulled into the area and drawn into the cells. The tissue that was dehydrated and stiff is immediately improved. In order to achieve this rehydration effect, you must maintain compression of a small, isolated area on the roller. Heavy, uncomfortable, or painful pressure should be avoided. If you Shear properly, you may feel areas of tenderness, but it shouldn't hurt. (Remember, pain is your signal to ease back pressure.)

Now let's try Rinsing.

Calf Rinse

▶ *Sit on the floor and place your arms behind you for support. With your right knee bent, rotate your right leg inward and place your inner ankle on the roller. Your foot is relaxed, and your big toe is close to the floor.*

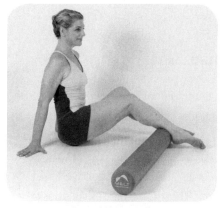

▶ *Lean forward and slowly straighten your right leg to allow the roller to move up your inner calf with consistent, light pressure. It's okay if the roller doesn't travel all the way up your calf.*

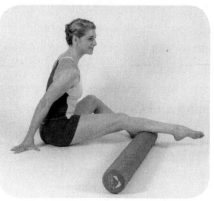

> *Rotate your leg so the back of your leg is on the roller.*

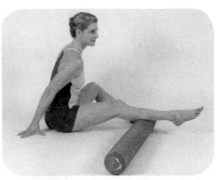

> *Lean back and slowly bend your knee to allow the roller to move down the back side of your calf with consistent, light pressure. Stop before your ankle and repeat the Rinse 3–4 times.*

> *Repeat on the other leg.*

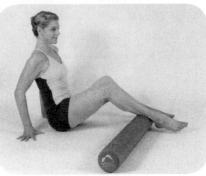

Rinse

The technique of Rinsing involves moving the connective tissue fluid in the specific directions that fluid flows in the body. This flushes the tissues with fluid in harmony with the tissue's natural energetic flow, or tensional energy, to create lasting results you will sense.

In order to MELT connective tissue, you must move slowly on the roller—don't be in a hurry. The important details about Rinsing are doing it in the right direction and keeping your pressure relatively light. Rinsing is a light, consistent sweep of the tissue just beneath the skin—much lighter than Gliding or Shearing. Rinsing is more about the consistency of light pressure you maintain than about the depth of pressure you apply. When and where you Rinse will be dependent on which MELT map you do.

Rinsing and Connective Tissue

Rinsing takes the new fluid production that Shearing stimulates in a small area and flushes the fluid through the tissues. When you Rinse, you help spread the fluid movement throughout the entire body. This creates the global rehydration effect, initiating the whole-body integration of hydration. Rinsing restores the cohesive fluid movement within the entire connective tissue system, which allows a full body balancing state to occur. The Autopilot relies on the fluid state of connective tissue to transport information quickly from head to toe for you to sustain efficient balance. Rinsing helps open this information highway so your Autopilot maintains a clear signal to your center of gravity and all your joints.

Because the connective tissue is a seamless system, you don't have to Rinse every area that you Glide and Shear. What's important is that you Rinse in the direction of the whole-body flow in the connective tissue system. I call this directional fluid flow tensional energy.

Tensional Energy

Through my hands-on practice, I have identified that there is a directional, continuous energetic life force in the body. I can feel this vibrational fluid movement with my hands. This energetic force moves in a constant flow, like a river, and has multidirectional current.

This perpetual, cyclical wave travels down the back side of the body and up the front. It returns back down the sides of the body and travels up again through the inside of the legs and the center of the body. The motion continues downward in a spiral loop around the body in a helix pattern and then back up again through the center of the body. This energetic current functions in an oppositional, or tensional, relationship, which allows the body to work with and against gravity so you can remain upright and stay grounded. There is no starting or ending place. This continuous force is not just energetic; it is physiologic. The Autopilot relies on this constant motion within the body to provide vibrational communication for its GPS system, but stuck stress interrupts, alters, and diverts tensional energy.

The tensional energy model informs and grounds many existing ancient and progressive healing modalities and creates a template for the discovery of new ones. You can benefit from the understanding of this highly responsive system to improve your own self-healing. The Gliding, Shearing, and Rinsing techniques and the MELT maps all work in the direction of tensional energy.

MELT Compression Tips and Precautions

Stay Stable

You must keep your core engaged while you Rehydrate so you remain stable. This also ensures that your arms, neck, shoulders, and legs aren't overburdened when you move your body over the roller and that you maintain the appropriate amount of body weight on the mass that is on the roller. This way, you will achieve the full benefits of the techniques. If you need additional support when doing the MELT compression techniques, consider using a bolster or yoga blocks to help you keep your body weight over the roller.

Pain Tolerance

Remember, you want to "wake up a little something" in the tissue, not overstimulate it or the sensory nervous system. Overstimulation can create inflammation and reduce the benefits of your self-treatment—and MELT is designed to reduce pain and inflammation, not increase it. In order to get the full benefits of MELT, it is important to listen to your body and make adjustments when (or ideally before) you feel pain. When you experience an intense sensation, pull back the amount of pressure you are applying and Shear more if needed.

Less Is Always More

The connective tissue responds to a specific amount of pressure applied in a precise manner. Applying too much pressure, moving too fast, and staying on an area too long actually decrease the benefits of MELT.

Do Not MELT the Spaces

Never Glide, Shear, or Rinse directly on any area of the body described as a space (belly, neck, etc.), as there are exposed nerves and organs in these areas that should only be treated by a specialist. Only MELT the masses—the spaces will benefit from the fluids you produce when you rehydrate the masses.

Focused Breath

As you Rehydrate, focus your breathing into the body part that you are compressing. Taking a focused breath stimulates the vital connection between the diaphragm and your nervous system to allow you to relax and ease into the compression. This focused breath also aids in circulating freshly oxygenated blood and fluids throughout the entire body. This helps to alleviate excess tension in other areas of your body so you can gain the maximum benefits of the compression techniques. Don't hold your breath when you compress!

▶ MELT Two-Directional Length Technique

Length involves moving two specific masses of the body, such as your hip and your heel, away from each other at the same pace to create tensional length in the connective tissue between them. Think of pulling on a rubber band in two opposing directions to make it taut. With your body, you are moving two bony masses in opposite directions and then holding that position and taking deep focused breaths while the tissue adapts.

To achieve the greatest rehydration effect, take time to really sense the tensional pull between the two focused parts of the body. Setting up the proper position is the key. To lengthen connective tissue, you must use specific muscles to align your joints in the proper position in order to get full contact with the tissue. Engaging your core muscles will help you gain stability and maintain the proper position.

In order to create Two-Directional Length, the details of how you use the roller and which body parts you move in opposition are different for each area. Detailed instructions are outlined in the MELT maps in Chapter 13.

MELT Length Tips and Precautions

Duration on Roller

The maximum amount of time you should lie lengthwise (along your spine) on the roller or have the roller on any mass—like the base of the skull or under the pelvis—is ten minutes. If you are pregnant, injured, or uncomfortable on the roller in any position, shorten the duration of compression to four minutes and build your time in one-minute increments every other time you MELT, until the maximum ten-minute duration is met.

Three-Breath Rule

Remember, less is more—get in and get out. Only hold any MELT length position for the amount of time equivalent to three deep, focused breaths. If you hold the position longer, you could cause your muscles to fatigue and send mixed messages from your body to your brain. You can always release the pull and repeat the technique a second time.

▶ MELT Length

Let's try lengthening the back of your leg from your hip to your heel.

Hip to Heel Press

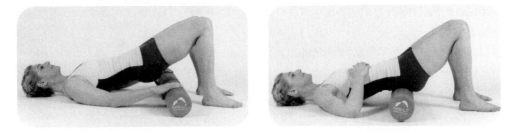

▶ *Lie on the floor, bend your knees, and put your feet flat on the floor, hip-width apart. Place the roller on the floor underneath your knees. Push your feet into the floor, lift up your hips, and position the roller under your pelvis (on the sacrum), just below the low back.*

To check if the roller is in the right place, draw both knees toward your chest. The roller should not feel like it's going to slip out. If it does, move the roller toward your low back. Nor should it feel like the roller is under your low back. If it does, move it down.

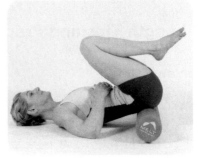

▶ *Place your left foot on the floor so your knee is in line with your hip. Raise your right thigh so your knee points toward the ceiling.*

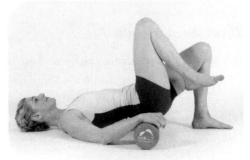

▶ *Straighten your right leg out in front of you and flex your ankle. Keep your pelvis heavy on top of the roller in a slight tilt, and your mid ribs relaxed and weighted to the floor.*

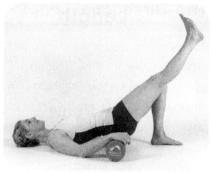

▶ *Keeping your leg straight, slowly bring your right flexed foot toward the ceiling and stop before your knee bends. (Keep the leg straight without locking or hyperextending the knee or creating pain in the knee.)*

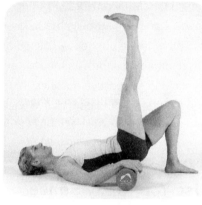

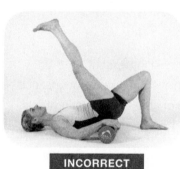

INCORRECT

Even if you are very flexible, don't extend your leg beyond a ninety-degree angle. If your leg is angled toward your nose, you will lose the ability to lengthen the connective tissue on the back of your leg.

▶ *On an exhale, in two directions, actively flex your ankle and tilt your pelvis, keeping your pelvis weighted to the top of the roller. Take a focused breath as you feel the tensional pull from your heel all the way down to your hip.*

▶ *Inhale and relax the foot. Then exhale and actively flex your foot and allow the pelvis to sink into the roller to find your tilt. Take a focused breath and pause as you accentuate the pull again. Repeat one more time on this side, then bring your right foot to the floor.*

▶ *Repeat on the other side.*

Two-Directional Length and Connective Tissue

Although connective tissue is flexible, its role is to manage tension and resist excessive stretch. The collagen fibers in the tissue resist in a protective, supportive way to reduce the potential of tearing in both muscles and connective tissue when you move—if the tissue is hydrated. Dehydration in the connective tissue causes poor extensibility and responsiveness of the tissue. It also hinders its role as the body's tensegrity architectural support system.

When you intentionally lengthen connective tissue to its end range, two-directionally, you can create a rehydration effect and restore the extensibility of the connective tissue. Lengthening pulls the fluid out of the connective tissue. When you let go, the receptors in the connective tissue are triggered to generate more fluid in the area.

Lengthening improves the resilience of the connective tissue and restores its elastic and supportive qualities. More space is created in the joints by rehydrating and lengthening the connective tissue, improving the integrity, stability, and alignment of the joints.

Use Your Body Sense

Although you will be using muscle to create the oppositional movement, your Body Sense will be your most important tool to effectively achieve the two-directional pull of your connective tissue. Learning to sense tensional pull of connective tissue versus muscular stretch takes practice and good Body Sense. Knowing the difference between the sensations is the key.

Two-directional tensional pull of connective tissue is felt in a longer line of the body, such as the entire back of your leg, than a stretch of muscle is, such as in your calf. Unlike an isolated muscle stretch, the pull always extends across and beyond a joint. With a muscular stretch, the pull is felt in a small region, usually close to and not beyond a joint. Remember, muscles can only stretch as far as connective tissue allows. The best time to stretch is after you do your MELT map. You will find that when you lengthen and rehydrate connective tissue, muscular flexibility dramatically improves—immediately.

If you feel a muscular stretch, you have extended beyond the proper length position, which inhibits your ability to stimulate connective tissue and achieve the hydration benefits. For example, lengthening the tissue on the entire back of the leg should not feel like a pull only in your calf. When this happens, reset your position and move more slowly to create the two-directional movement to sense the light tug in the connective tissue in a longer line down the back of the leg. Although the pull may feel less intense than a muscle stretch, the benefits to the muscle and the connective tissue are far greater and longer lasting. If you find you cannot reach the proper position, try doing the compression techniques in that area first. Then try the length position again and see if you can achieve the two-directional length.

Lengthening takes practice. Soon you will find it easy to obtain and sense the proper position and create immediate results.

Comparing Length as an Assessment Technique

In a MELT map, sometimes you will use a MELT length technique to assess imbalances in a particular area of your body. To do this, do the same length technique before and after doing the compression technique on the same area of the body and see if you feel a difference. For example, you might do Rib Length, then Glide, Shear, and Rinse your Upper Back, and then repeat Rib Length. The second time you perform Rib Length, your ability to extend should improve.

As you perform each lengthening technique, also pay attention to whether one side needs more length or feels more restricted than the other. To address this imbalance, you can repeat the MELT length technique on that side. You may even want to repeat the MELT compression techniques for that area of the body before repeating the length technique.

Mass Stability and Differentiation

During upper body length techniques, you will be focusing on keeping your ribs and pelvis, or the primary masses, heavy and stable while creating the two-directional movements. During lower body length techniques, you will need to differentiate movement of one mass while keeping the other stable. For example, to get the most out of the Hip to Heel Press, you will keep your ribs heavy to the floor while you sink your pelvis on top of the roller.

Focused Breath

Take a focused breath by putting your intention on breathing into the area you are lengthening. When you take slow, focused breaths into the regions you are MELTing, your inhalation deepens the tensional pull while your exhale supports the Reflexive Core. This allows you to gain the full benefit of the specific MELT length move.

Body Changes: After completing the MELT Rehydration techniques, you may notice these specific changes when you Reassess:

- Your masses feel fuller and weighted to the floor.

- Fluid movement is restored in the entire body.

- Your body feels closer to the reference point of ideal alignment.

8

Release

One day, while trying to find a way to manipulate the base of my skull to release the joints in my neck, I started experimenting with homemade tools to simulate what worked with my clients. The tool that seemed to work best was a piece of PVC piping wrapped in bubble wrap and a yoga mat, held together with duct tape. With the base of my skull on the contraption, I slowly adjusted my body weight, the pressure and position of my skull, and the location of this homemade roller to see what might work. I moved and adjusted my position as I would do to my clients with my hands. When I reassessed, my neck felt totally open and relaxed. It was easier to turn my head from side to side, and I could breathe easier too. I couldn't believe it. I had actually decompressed my own neck. I felt amazing the entire day. The next day I tried it again and got the same effect. It seemed like a miracle that I could decompress, or release, the tension in my neck and my own cervical vertebrae and sense a notable change the entire day. The movement and pressure I used were very subtle, replicating what I do using my hands-on techniques.

I was excited to share my new trick with Lynn, my client with severe neck and TMJ. TMJ is a condition in which the jaw doesn't align correctly. The jaw can become so stiff that it is difficult to open the mouth to a normal degree. TMJ can cause extreme jaw pain and headaches, as it did for Lynn. When I told her about my release discovery, she said, "Do you think it would help me?" Decompressing her neck with my hands always gave her great relief in her jaw and progressively decreased her head and neck tension. I told her we could spend a little time and try the new release technique at the end of the session.

When her session time was almost over, I had purposefully omitted decompressing her neck with my hands. I had her do the Rest Assess on the floor. I asked her to pay particular attention to how her neck and jaw felt. I handed her my PVC contraption and talked her through what I had done to myself. When she reassessed, she took a deep breath, yawned, popped her eyes wide open, and said, "Holy cow! Did you see how wide I just opened my jaw to yawn?! My jaw didn't even click. I think it really worked, Sue!"

I sent her home with my little homemade tool and instructions to repeat the technique every day until our next appointment. Whenever I decompressed her neck with my hands, her jaw pain usually went away for three to five days. This time, she came back the following week saying, "My jaw is seriously better. I don't want to say it out loud because I'm afraid I might jinx it. My jaw still feels like it did when I walked out of your office last week."

She went on, "I actually think it's gotten a little better each day. It made my jaw feel better almost every time I did it, and I haven't had one single headache, either. The day before yesterday, I slept for eight hours straight for the first time in a long while, and I woke up feeling rested. I realized my jaw didn't click when I ate breakfast this morning. I think it may have been like that since earlier this week."

Her face looked totally relaxed. I could see that she also looked younger and more vibrant, her skin and eyes looked clear, and her energy level appeared to be the best I had ever seen it.

"You are totally onto something here, Sue. Now if you can figure out a way to do that same thing for my husband's snoring and back pain, you might even save my marriage!" Lynn said with a laugh and a smile.

I was amazed and excited. If Lynn could decompress her neck, so could my other clients. But that wasn't all. Now I had to figure out how to decompress my low back on my own. I had seen so many clients who needed this. According to the University of Arizona College of Medicine, 80 percent of adults experience low back pain in their lifetime, and it is the most common type of chronic pain. Neck pain is number two. The reason is that as the two largest spaces of the body, the neck and low back are the most challenged during our day-to-day movement. As a result, the spine in these areas is the most susceptible to excess compression and torque. Chronic pain, inflammation, and joint damage follow. This creates a domino effect that begins with aches and stiffness and leads to common health issues such as headaches, insomnia, digestive problems, and injuries. Accelerated aging and chronic health problems can follow, leaving you with limited treatment options including medicine, surgery, and a more sedentary lifestyle—incomplete solutions that carry risks of their own.

As I developed more decompression techniques, I shared them with my clients over the course of a year. The feedback I received was astounding. Even clients who had other issues, like knee pain or digestive distress, started feeling as if these symptoms lessened as they continued to decompress their own spine. It seemed I had created a technique that I could teach people to do on their own to get out of pain and stay out. The decompression techniques created some of the most noticeable, powerful changes in all of MELT.

Initially, the MELT instructors and I only showed these techniques to our one-on-one clients.

I was reluctant to show people in a group fitness environment a subtle technique that, at the time, took at least a few minutes to explain and set up and then another five minutes to actually perform. I was still trying to make the concept of MELT seem like it was solely working toward the primary fitness goal of improving performance. Getting out of pain was just a side effect that people were experiencing, not what I was asserting that MELT might be able to do. That idea seemed far too therapeutic for the fitness world I'd been a part of for so many years.

As I refined the other MELT techniques in group classes and people were seeing overwhelming results, I could still see the need for decompression techniques. With time, practice, and patience along with getting to know my students who returned to class week after week, I learned how to simplify the language and cueing of decompression, and I found the right recipe for Gliding and Shearing prior to releasing. Ultimately, I learned how to teach room after room of people to understand and feel what it was like to decompress their own neck and low back spaces. As more and more people filled the room, I would frequently find myself saying, "I get paid a lot of money to decompress people's neck and low back with my hands. What is far more rewarding for me is to show someone how to do it for themselves so they can get out of pain and stay out. Now you can do it on your own too. You're welcome." It was then that I realized my private practice had grown far beyond the walls of my office space!

▶ The Basics of Decompression

Decompressing your neck and low back, as well as the joints of your spine, hands, and feet, is essential for anyone to live pain-free. MELT gives you the tools to release joint compression.

Find Some Space

No one ever complains about getting taller as they get older. That's because as you age, you shrink from the loss of space in the collective joints of your body. Repetitive movements and postures, as well as gravity, take a toll on your body's ability to maintain the vital space within your joints. This doesn't only affect people who are getting along in years. If you've ever experienced neck or low back pain, difficulty turning your neck, or stiffness in your low back, you've experienced a loss of space. Along with the hands and the feet, the areas that are usually affected first are the neck and abdomen/low back space, or the "primary body spaces." These spaces, like joints, are what allow you to bend, turn, and move without your masses damaging organs and nerves. Imagine if your ribs extended down to your pelvis—you wouldn't be able to bend over! The primary spaces are important.

Regardless of what causes the loss of space in your neck or low back, the result is the same—the bones of your spine come closer together. When the vertebrae compress, the disks in between and the nerves that emerge from the spinal column also become compressed. When nerves are compressed, pinched, and irritated, you feel pain. Before now, pain was the first sign of chronic compression.

When you have pain caused by compression, that's a sign that you also have connective tissue inflammation, which leads to joint damage. Pain and tingling originating from the compressed nerves in the spine can be sensed in other areas of the body, which is known as referred pain. Sensory and motor communication becomes impaired and delayed, and the spine becomes more misaligned. Your Autopilot has to work harder just to maintain a misaligned posture.

When the spine is compressed, you lose some or all of the natural curve in your neck and low back. With less balance in the curves, your spine loses the shock absorption and buoyancy it needs to help you move with ease, without compression or compensation. In this less than ideal alignment, joints become fixed, and disk damage and injury can follow. Misalignment spreads to the "secondary body spaces," such as your shoulders and knees, and the cycle of compression, pain, inflammation, and joint damage starts all over again. Without regaining the integrity and stability in the curves and the space in your neck and low back, misalignments and compression in these secondary spaces will always return.

Whether the compression has been occurring for months, years, or decades, you can regain lost space by regularly releasing compression in the neck and low back with MELT decompression techniques. The first time you try the techniques, you will feel immediate changes in your alignment, and you'll be on your way to being pain-free.

▶ MELT Decompression Techniques

In this section, you are going to learn how to decompress your neck. Always assess before you decompress your neck. You will then use the Shearing techniques to bring fresh fluid to the area for the greatest decompression effect. Keep your ribs stable and still as you move the neck during the decompression techniques.

Neck Release Sequence

Neck Turn Assess

Base of Skull Shear

Neck Decompress

Neck Turn Reassess

Neck Turn Assess

▸ *Lie on your back with your legs extended. You can bend your knees if lying with your legs straight causes unnecessary tension in your back. Be comfortable as you assess.*

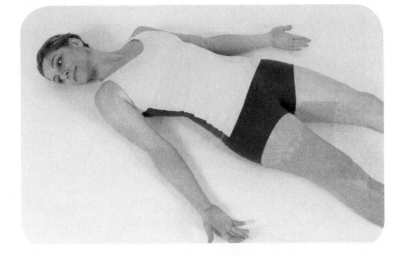

▸ *Use your Body Sense to notice the curve of your neck. Without touching your neck, notice the shape and size of your neck space. Ideally, the highest point of the neck curve is closer to your head than to your shoulders.*

▸ *Slowly turn your head to the right and then to the left, keeping your chin away from your shoulders. Do you feel like you're able to turn your head more in either direction? Do you feel any pain or tension? Does it feel like your shoulders move when you turn your head?*

▸ *Take note of what you feel so you can compare after you Release your neck.*

Base of Skull Shear

▶ *Lie on your right side and rest the base of your skull, just behind your ear, on the top of the roller. Bend your knees and reach your right arm out so your shoulders are relaxed.*

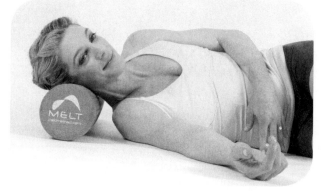

▶ *Take a focused breath and begin creating small head circles in either direction 5–6 times to Shear the base of your skull. Then pause for a moment, take a focused breath, and allow this area to sink further into the roller.*

▶ *Open your left knee toward the ceiling so you're lying on the right half of your back. The roller is still under the base of your skull on the right side, an inch or so away from your ear, closer to the center of the base of your skull.*

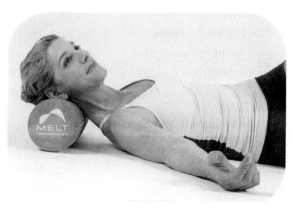

▶ *Take a focused breath and repeat the circles to Shear. Pause and take a focused breath.*

▶ *Turn onto your left side and repeat the Shear on the left side. In each spot, pause and take a focused breath.*

▶ *Lie on your back with your knees bent and rest the center of the base of your skull on the roller. Lift your chin slightly.*

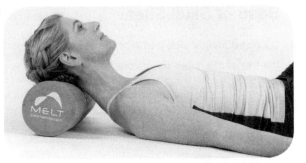

▶ *While maintaining consistent pressure, create small figure eight motions on the center of the base of your skull 5–6 times.*
Keep your pressure constant and your chin slightly lifted. Pause and take a focused breath.

Neck Decompress

▶ *Keep your knees bent, place your hands on the roller, and push the roller up about 1 inch toward the center of the back of your head. Take your hands away from the roller. Tip your nose toward the ceiling and apply gentle pressure on top of the roller. You must maintain consistent pressure throughout this move.*

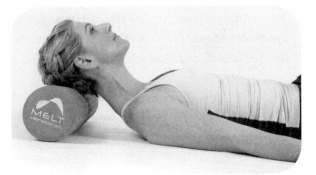

▶ *Inhale and, on an exhale, slowly nod your chin down slightly.*

▶ *Inhale as you hold this position and, on the exhale, lift your chin slightly and return your nose toward the ceiling. Pause on the inhale; move on the exhale.*

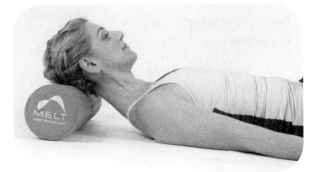

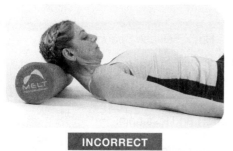

You are not trying to touch your chin to your chest. The movement you create should be small and slow. Notice if your shoulders lift as you tip your head upward. Keep your upper back still and relaxed.

▶ *Repeat this head nod 4 times, pausing on the inhale, moving on the exhale.*

▶ *Remove the roller from the back of your head and gently bring your head to the floor.*

Neck Turn Reassess

▶ *Lie on your back with your legs extended. Bend your knees if your back is uncomfortable.*

▶ *Sense the curve of your neck. Does it feel lighter? Do you notice a more distinct curve just below the base of the skull?*

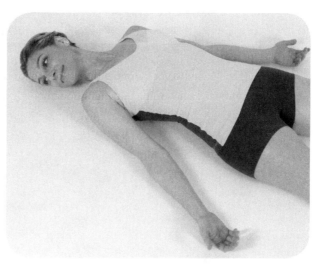

▶ *Turn your head slowly from left to right. Do you have more range of motion? Is there less pain or stiffness in your neck? Are your back and shoulders more relaxed as you turn your head?*

▶ *If you sense any of these changes, you have decompressed your neck.*

Body Changes: After completing the Neck Release Sequence, you may notice these specific changes when you Reassess:

- Your neck curve feels more lifted near the skull.

- Neck turning has greater range with less effort and less pain.

- You may feel like you're turning your head from higher in your neck.

9

The Hand and Foot Treatment

When word got out that I was helping all kinds of people leave their pain behind, my practice suddenly went from nine or ten clients a week to forty. It was an amazing time. In each session, I was doing a mix of hands-on therapy and teaching clients how to self-treat with MELT and the roller.

One morning, a shocking thing happened to me. I went to grab a glass from the cabinet, and it slipped out of my hand. When I went to pick it up, it happened again. I tried to make a fist and realized I had almost completely lost my grip. At first, I shook out my hands and assumed it would pass. I thought I must have slept on it wrong. It didn't go away. I tried to massage my own hands, but I literally wasn't able to. Using your hands to try to massage your hands when they're not working . . . well, doesn't work. An hour passed with no change. I canceled all my clients for the day and immediately went into my office to see what I could use to work on my hands without using my hands. Unknowingly, this was the day I began developing the MELT Hand and Foot Treatment.

I didn't have the right-size tools, so I went to a local toy store and bought different types of balls. I bought Kadima balls, super balls, and jack balls. I even pulled a few oval rocks from the potted plants on my balcony and started trying to simulate various techniques. I had learned the importance of assessment, so the first thing I did was assess my grip by clenching a ball in my fist. My grip in both hands was pretty weak, even in my dominant hand. This is when I began to realize that the repetition of working on clients with my hands was affecting me in ways I hadn't recognized.

I was very familiar with working on people's hands. Usually it was because they had arthritis, carpal tunnel, tennis elbow, or disorders that directly affected the neurological control of their hands. I was surprised to realize that I needed the same type of treatment. I started playing around with the balls to replicate the hands-on techniques I use on my clients. Not all of the manual therapies I use on my clients are possible with an inanimate object, so I started with the ones that were. I tried some Gliding and Shearing, just like I would do with the roller. I experimented with different ways to mobilize the joints in my hands and fingers using the concepts of Kerry J. D'Ambrogio's manual therapy technique, Positional Release Therapy. When I Rinsed, I instinctively pressed the ball all the way up my forearm. When I reassessed my grip, it had noticeably improved and was more equal in both hands.

The next morning when I woke up, I was relieved to find that I still had a more solid grip and only slight stiffness in my wrists. I immediately repeated what I had done with the balls the day before. I felt ready to see clients again. As I worked on my first client of the day, I could sense that something amazing was happening. My ability to use my hands to assess and treat was better than ever. My Body Sense in my hands was heightened, and this continued throughout the day.

Self-treating my hands became part of my morning routine. I also began to notice that my neck felt better at the end of a day, before I even got on the roller. This made complete sense as I had long seen the correlation between neck and hand issues in my clients. My face even started to look more relaxed. Over the following months, I tracked my progress as I used the balls in different ways. Because the hands have so many joints so close together, I knew it was important to find the best way to create positive compression and yield the greatest change.

I was ready to show some clients this new technique, and I had many eager volunteers. I quickly realized that it was better to start people off with only a soft ball, instead of sending them home with all the balls. My clients with arthritis and other hand issues had little to no fluid available around their joints to begin with. We had to move slowly and for less time to first generate fluid and then get the fluid moving. Without the fluid present, the firmer balls and compression could increase irritation and inflammation.

The results were rather staggering. Clients who had chronic hand or wrist pain were seeing immediate results. They sensed greater ease of movement, increased grip strength, and reduction of pain, swelling, and inflammation. Many said their necks felt better, just like mine had. Eventually, clients were asking me if their improvements in sleep, headaches, migraines, and sinus issues could be attributed to the Hand

Treatment. Clients with lung and breathing issues, including asthma, were experiencing dramatic improvements in their chronic symptoms as well.

I was astounded by how this simple Hand Treatment was able to restore my clients' hope and well-being. I was accustomed to giving my clients homework that they usually never did. I was always encouraging them to make simple lifestyle changes that would make them feel better. Instead, they would rather come see me so I would "fix" them. However, these same clients were suddenly motivated and empowered to take care of themselves in ways I had never seen. They were improving their own aging process, and they could tell. This made me want to share the Hand Treatment with more people.

▶ My Final Discovery

As I was teaching people the Hand Treatment, I started experimenting with using the balls on my feet. I had many clients with foot issues such as bunions, chronic foot pain and swelling, plantar fasciitis, and neuromas. I knew that if they could self-treat their feet between our sessions, it could make a huge difference in their pain, inflammation, and swelling.

I was also excited by the idea that I might have a solution to one of my occupational hazards—touching people's feet. Not that I have anything against feet. Some of my clients have immaculately pedicured feet. However, many do not. Feet in New York City are transportation, which means New Yorkers' feet, mine included, get a workout whenever we leave home. This produces sweaty, stinky feet, and during summer flip-flop weather, they also get dirty. Add bunions, warts, athlete's foot, fungal nails, calluses, and other foot issues and you can see why it's not my favorite part of the job.

The hands and the feet have a lot in common. They both have thousands of proprioceptors and sensory nerve endings and an abundance of joints. Indeed, proprioceptors exist in the highest concentration closest to the joints. There are also structural similarities between the hands and the feet, so it made sense to start by applying what worked on my hands to my feet. The results I experienced were more powerful and immediate than any I had achieved before. At the time, I was MELTing with the roller every day, so I was very surprised that the big changes I experienced were in my *body* when I was treating my *feet*.

When I did the Foot Treatment, my low back instantly felt more open and my spine was more flexible. For the first time in years, I could squat down to the floor without hearing my knees make a popping or cracking sound. My breathing felt more expansive. I felt calmer and more grounded. I had more energy during my workouts, and my recovery time afterward was significantly reduced.

I was astounded. I started MELTing with the roller less so I could better identify the specific changes I was making with the Foot Treatment. I found that when I would MELT my feet, the self-treatments with the roller lasted longer. At this point it seemed insane that the feet weren't one of the first areas of the body I had tried self-treatment on. In my hands-on work, grounding the body through the feet was always a primary focus. In hindsight, it seems obvious: work on the feet to ground the body and help the Autopilot find the center of gravity before working anywhere else.

I tried doing all the techniques on one foot before doing the other so I could compare the changes in my body from side to side. After I did the Foot Treatment on one side, I reassessed by closing my eyes and using my Body Sense to feel any differences. The foot that I had done the treatment on felt cushioned and firmly grounded on the floor. This is when I really started to get a sense of what groundedness felt like. It was as if I were standing on memory foam or sand instead of a hard floor. The leg on that same side felt more cohesive, grounded, and yet lighter.

On the other leg, I noticed the joints, and my leg felt heavier. My foot felt ungrounded, as if it were just hovering on the ground. I began the Foot Treatment on the opposite side the next time to see if the changes were similar and as obvious—and they were. I began to document my results.

I started doing additional side-to-side comparative assessments. I did a spine flex assessment after treating one foot.

I compared my arm reach and noticed that the arm on the treated side of my body would reach longer—sometimes by inches. This indicated that stimulating my feet was driving the fluid through my spine all the way to my fingertips. When I bent over to touch my toes, I felt more flexible in my spine and legs on the side that I had treated. There was less tightness and tension. It felt like I had done a big stretching session on one leg when I had only done the MELT techniques with balls under my foot. After doing the treatment on both feet, I could sense that my stride felt longer and lighter when I walked. I seemed to move with greater ease and felt less clunky. All these changes were even more pronounced if I drank water before I did the Foot Treatment.

When I started introducing the Foot Treatment to my clients, they saw the same changes that I had—and even more. I learned more by being able to observe the changes in my clients. It was becoming clear to me that the Foot Treatment was enhancing the body's system of effortless, upright stability. I observed that my clients' grounding, stability, balance, and flexibility improved.

I started having my clients do a standing Autopilot Assess before and after they treated their feet. It was very clear that their Autopilot could more easily find their center of gravity after the Foot Treatment. I came to see that there was a system of the body that was designed to stabilize the spine and keep the whole body upright, which ultimately helped me simplify and articulate the Rooted Core component of the NeuroCore model. I learned that the mechanism of the Rooted Core's head-to-toe stability system could be directly accessed through the feet just as the Reflexive Core could be accessed through the diaphragm while the spine is stimulated by the roller.

▶ The Perfect Combination of Techniques and Balls

I continued to refine the assessments, techniques, and sequences to yield the greatest results. One of the techniques that I spent the most time thinking about and researching was Position Point Pressing. Initially, my intention for including this technique was just to mobilize the joints and rebalance the arches. When I shared the Foot Treatment with my clients, I realized that stimulating these points was also creating positive changes in digestion, sleep, anxiety, and a host of chronic symptoms that they previously only felt relief from whenever they had a session with me.

I had my theories, but I wanted research that could explain what I was doing. Do reflexology, acupuncture, and acupressure use these same points? Were these position points accessing the body's meridians? In some cases yes, and in some no. I came to realize that the points I had determined to be the most beneficial were the "end points" of the fascial connections of Tom Myers's myofascial meridian model. (Since then, studies have shown that the acupuncture meridians correlate with these connective tissue meridians.) By stimulating these points, I was simultaneously mobilizing the joints, rejuvenating hydration in the connective tissue, heightening Body Sense, stimulating the sensory nerve endings, and energizing the connective tissue meridians. Then Gliding, Shearing, and Rinsing were providing further rehydration.

Because your feet (and hands) are at the ends of your body, connective tissue fluid and blood tends to accumulate in these areas. So I added an additional technique called Friction, which creates light stimulation to encourage any stagnant blood flow in connective tissue to be returned through the body in the lymphatic system.

The techniques of the Hand and Foot Treatment collectively Reconnect, Rebalance, Rehydrate, and Release to create change throughout the whole body. That's why I refer to this treatment as a global technique. Even though you are stimulating only your hands and feet, you are making profound changes in your entire body.

Given that the Hand and Foot Treatment simulates what I do with my hands, fingers, and elbows as a hands-on practitioner, I had to spend a lot of time making sure the equipment was just right. I chose to make four different balls—one large and soft, one large and firm, one small and soft, and another small and firm. These sizes and densities are specifically designed for the MELT Hand and Foot Treatment. Not only will you get the best results using these balls, but you'll also be guaranteed not to expose yourself to toxic chemicals or dyes, latex, or phthalates.

(The MELT Hand and Foot Treatment Kit—including eight balls, a bunion band, and two illustrated guides in a convenient travel case—is available at www.meltmethod.com. The Hand and Foot Treatment DVD and MELT Method DVD are also available on the website.)

The large soft ball is the most gentle, and it can be used for all of the Hand and Foot Treatment techniques. You will use the large soft ball to get started. If you want to use the other balls, refer to the instructions in the kit and the DVD.

▶ The MELT Hand and Foot Treatment

In just minutes, you can self-treat your hands or feet and achieve all Four R's—Reconnect, Rebalance, Rehydrate, and Release. The Hand and Foot Treatment is a global technique that provides whole-body rejuvenation.

The Hand and Foot Treatment techniques erase the negative effects of daily wear and tear on your hands and feet and improve your whole body's overall alignment, connection, and flexibility by using specialized self-treatment balls. These quick self-care techniques can easily be done anywhere by anyone.

Everyday life is hard on your hands. The MELT Hand Treatment relieves the stiffness brought on by repetitive daily activities that's felt as pain in your hands and wrists and, over time, as chronic neck, shoulder, and back aches. And every day, with every step you take, your feet bear your entire body weight. The more active you are, the greater the impact on your feet. The MELT Foot Treatment relieves common foot pain and problems, and alleviates tension in the low back and spine.

The MELT Hand and Foot Treatment helps to keep your hands and feet more flexible and helps restore whole-body mobility, balance, and stability. Many people report an overall feeling of well-being and body ease after MELTing. Best of all, the benefits you experience often continue long after you MELT.

❱ MELT Hand and Foot Techniques

The MELT Hand and Foot Treatment uses five techniques to create whole-body changes:

Position Point Pressing applies direct, tolerable pressure to specific points of the hands and feet to mobilize the joints and rejuvenate them with essential fluid. Position Point Pressing improves not only the mobility of the hands and feet but also the neurological connection between your extremities and every other system in your body.

Glide, Shear, and Rinse techniques are used to activate and restore the hydration of the connective tissue in your hands and feet, just as they do for your body. As an added benefit, when you Rinse your hands and feet it helps to relieve tension in the neck and low back.

Friction involves rubbing the ball in light, random directions to stimulate the most superficial layer of connective tissue and encourage fluid movement in the lymphatic system. You can even do Friction on its own anytime during the day to stimulate your lymph system. This helps to reduce inflammation in the hands and feet, so you always want to end with this technique. Go for a light, superficial pressure. This technique creates the same effect as putting your joints next to hot tub jets. If the pressure is too heavy, you won't achieve the proper results.

As with the body, the MELT protocol of Reconnecting before and after each sequence or treatment is important to achieving lasting change with the Hand and

Foot Treatment. Evaluating your body before and after your self-treatment will help you get a sense of the changes you're creating and will assist you in maintaining the results you achieve.

Hand and Foot Treatment Tips and Precautions

Breathing

As you MELT the hands and feet, focus your breath into the point you're compressing with the ball. This sends a message to the nervous system and triggers the rehydration effect. This will also heighten your Body Sense.

Pain Tolerance

When you begin MELTing, you may be surprised at how tender your hands and feet are. If you find an area of discomfort, that's your cue to ease back the pressure and breathe. Pain is always a signal that you are overdoing it and decreasing the desired effect. Remember: the balls are inanimate objects; they cannot hurt you—only you can hurt yourself with the balls. Whatever the pressure you think you should use, the ideal pressure will most likely be even lighter!

In this section, you are going to start with a Mini Soft Ball Hand and Foot Treatment. The more you MELT your hands and feet, the easier it will be—and you'll experience lasting results throughout your whole body.

Modifications

If you have injuries or issues such as a stress fracture, plantar fasciitis, or neuromas, MELT around the injury to rehydrate the tissue so you support healing without causing further irritation. You'll know you're ready to do the techniques directly on the area of concern when you can put pressure on the ball without pain. Pain is always your indication to ease off pressure or MELT around the area until your body lets you know it's ready.

If you have issues or conditions such as Dupuytren's, scleroderma, or rheumatoid arthritis, spend less time on each technique when you first begin doing the treatment. It will be especially important for you to drink plenty of water before and after you MELT.

▶ Mini Soft Ball Hand Treatment

Before You Begin

- These techniques can be done standing or seated at a table or desk, or sitting on the floor. You can also lie on your side to do the techniques, if that's more comfortable.

- Take off any rings, bracelets, and watches.

- Keep your upper body relaxed. Don't tense up your shoulders.

- Maintain a tolerable pressure. Don't put your full body weight on the balls.

As you complete this assessment, remember what you find and how your body feels. After you MELT, you will do this assessment again to sense and evaluate the changes that MELT has created.

Grip Assess

▶ *Place a soft ball in one hand and squeeze it 3–4 times as firmly as you can.*

▶ *Then place the ball in the other hand and notice whether your grip feels equal in strength or if you have a stronger grip in one hand than in the other. Remember how this feels.*

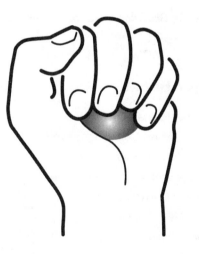

Glide

▶ *Place the soft ball on a table or other flat surface.*

▶ *On your right hand, with your palm down, Glide the ball from point 3 across the base of the palm to point 5 and return to point 3 with consistent pressure. Keep the tip of your middle finger on the table or floor as you create the Glide. Continue back and forth as you take 3–4 focused breaths.*

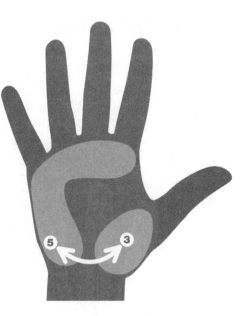

Shear

▶ *Place the soft ball under point 3, the thumb pad, on your right hand and create small circles as you take 3–4 focused breaths. Move slowly and take your time with Shearing the thumb pad, as this area often carries a lot of stuck stress.*

▶ *Repeat the Glide and Shear on the left hand.*

Finger Rinse

▶ *Place your left hand flat on the floor or a table. Use the right hand to rub the soft ball over the top of and in between each finger of the left hand in one direction, from the knuckle to the nail. (This also stimulates point 4 on the top hand, rehydrating the tissues of the wrist, reducing inflammation, and relieving wrist pain.)*

▶ *Repeat on the other hand.*

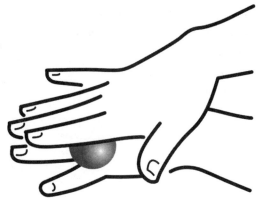

Friction

▶ *Using light, quick, random movements, rub one hand over the soft ball in a scribble-like motion. Be sure to include your fingers and wrists.*

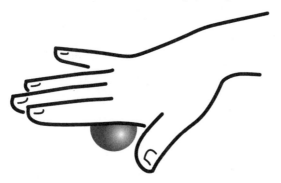

▶ *Repeat on the other hand.*

Grip Reassess

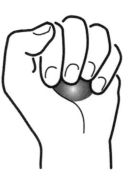

▶ *Remember what your grip strength felt like when you began and repeat the Grip Assess. Place the soft ball in one hand and squeeze it 3–4 times as firmly as you can. Repeat with the other hand. Can you now create a more powerful grip with less effort? Does your grip feel more equal from left to right?*

Body Changes: After completing the Hand Treatment, you may notice these specific changes when you Reassess:

• Neck, head, and shoulder tension is reduced.

• Tension and tightness in finger and wrist joints are released.

• Your hands feel more flexible and light.

THE HAND AND FOOT TREATMENT

▶ Mini Soft Ball Foot Treatment

Before You Begin

- As you do the treatment, stand with your feet directly below your hips and maintain an upright posture. Try to keep your head up and not look at your feet during the treatment. Instead, use your Body Sense to feel if you have the ball in the right spot under your foot.

- You can stand next to a wall or a chair to help you balance, if necessary. If standing is difficult, you can sit to do the Foot Treatment.

- Keep the pressure tolerable. You don't need to put your full body weight on the ball. If you feel pain, apply less pressure.

As you complete this assessment, remember how your body feels and reacts. After you MELT, you will do this assessment again to sense and evaluate the changes that MELT has created.

Body Scan Assess

▶ *Stand with your feet side by side, hip-width apart (approximately 6 inches). Close your eyes and use your Body Sense to notice your feet. Does it feel like you have more weight on your left or right side? Are you sensing that your weight is concentrated on a particular region of your feet?*

▶ *Use your Body Sense to scan up your legs. Notice the joints of your ankles, knees, and hips. Notice your muscles. Are your legs tense? Do you feel like you are using a lot of muscles to stand? Are your thigh and butt muscles engaged? See if you can relax these muscles and still remain comfortably standing. If so, this is how you know you are working too hard to simply stand up.*

Position Point Pressing

▌ *Stand up straight with your feet hip-width apart. Place the soft ball on the floor in front of you and step onto it with your right foot so the ball aligns with position point 1.*

▌ *Put your feet side by side and gently shift some of your body weight onto the ball to create tolerable pressure. Then shift some of your weight off the ball.*

▌ *Repeat this shifting 2–3 times to ease into tolerable compression while you take focused breaths.*

▌ *Step backward with the opposite foot and shift your weight to that foot.*

▌ *Place the ball under position point 5, in front of the heel bone. Apply tolerable compression to that point as you take a focused breath.*

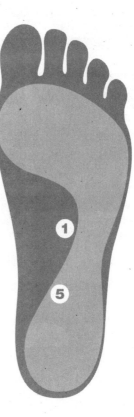

Glide

▌ *Place the ball on point 5, right in front of the heel. The ball of your foot and your toes are on the floor. Your heel is off the ground.*

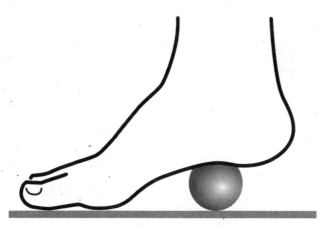

- *Keeping the front of your foot on the floor, slowly move the ball from side to side in front of the heel.*

- *Continue Gliding the ball from side to side as you work your way to the back of the heel and then back to point 5.*

Shear

- *With the ball on point 5, use a slightly heavier compression to wiggle your foot left to right. The ball should barely move.*

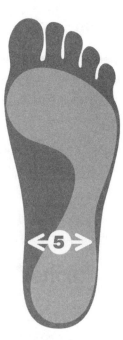

Rinse

- *Place the ball on point 2, directly under the big toe knuckle. Press the ball toward your heel in a continuous motion with tolerable, consistent pressure. For the greatest result, begin your Rinse with your foot slightly behind you so you can easily create a smooth toe-to-heel Rinse.*

- *Lift your foot, place the ball under the next knuckle, and Rinse.*

   Only Rinse in one direction.

- *Repeat for all five knuckles.*

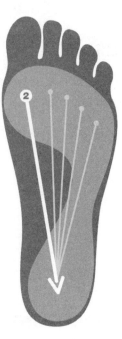

Friction

- *Using light, quick, random movements, rub your foot and toes over the ball in a scribble-like motion.*

Body Scan Reassess

▶ *Close your eyes and use your Body Sense to notice the side of the body you just self-treated. Notice your foot. Does it feel different than the other foot? (Not a big surprise—you've been rubbing your foot with a ball.)*

▶ *Notice the joints of your leg. You may find that you don't sense the leg as separate parts anymore, and instead your leg feels more cohesive. Notice if you feel more grounded.*

Now repeat all of the techniques on the other foot.

Final Body Scan Reassess

▶ *Close your eyes and use your Body Sense to feel your feet on the floor. Notice your joints. Do your legs feel more cohesive on both sides now? Do you feel more evenly grounded?*

Body Changes: After completing the Foot Treatment, you may notice these specific changes when you Reassess:

- Foot, knee, hip, and low back pain and tension are reduced.

- Feet and legs feel lighter and more flexible.

- Whole-body balance and stability are improved as the Autopilot regains its GPS signal to the center of gravity.

- Foot arches are rebalanced, and their buoyancy is enhanced.

Part
Three

10

Getting Started with Your MELT Practice

Your MELT self-treatment plan is a step-by-step guide to transforming your health. The first week, you will start with the Rebalance Sequence and the Hand and Foot Treatment. These sequences will help heighten your Body Sense, Reconnect you to your Autopilot, and Rebalance your NeuroCore. You will restore greater movement of your diaphragm, ground your body, and improve your body's tensional energy. I recommend starting by doing each sequence two to three times in the first week, but MELT is gentle enough that you can do any of these sequences every day. If you are or have recently been under a doctor's care, pay special attention to Chapter 14 for guidelines.

Next you will add the Upper and Lower Body Compression and Length Sequences to directly address stuck stress through rehydration of your connective tissue system. Then your body will be prepared to add the Release sequences so you can create more space in your neck and low back. You will continue to do the Hand and Foot Treatment a few times each week.

At this point, you will be ready to combine the sequences into MELT maps that address the four systemic effects of stuck stress. You will be familiar with the sequences and be able to maintain the changes you've made with shorter, ten-minute MELT sessions. There are also fifteen- to twenty-minute maps for when you have more time, and you can always return to your Upper and Lower Body Map for a full MELT session. I recommend doing this once a week (or more).

You are working your way toward MELTing for ten minutes, three times a week. Remember, you've never done Hands-Off Bodywork before. There will be a learning curve as you add each new sequence, so give yourself time to learn the moves. This is one time when "more is better." Once you become familiar with the moves and sequences, you will be able to MELT without even picking up this book!

▶ Getting Started Self-Treatment Plan

Here's an overview of your Getting Started Self-Treatment Plan: your first week of MELTing you will be doing the Soft Ball Hand and Foot Treatment and the Rebalance Sequence found in this chapter. These are the foundational components of MELT and the best place for you to start your journey into self-treatment. You will continue to do these when you learn the Upper and Lower Body Compression and Length Sequences in Chapter 11 and the Neck Release and Low Back Release Sequences in Chapter 12. In four to five weeks, you will have learned all of the basic MELT moves and be ready to do ten-, fifteen-, and twenty-minute MELT maps. The Hand Treatment, Foot Treatment, or the Rebalance Sequence are a part of every MELT map.

▶ Before You Begin

Here are pointers and precautions to keep in mind as you MELT for the first time.

When Should I MELT?

When you first begin, it's best to MELT at the end of your day, up to an hour before bedtime, especially if you have chronic pain. This way, you boost your body's healing mechanism and restore regulator so your sleep is more restful. Your Autopilot gets an opportunity to recover and recharge, and you get more benefits from your MELT session.

If you don't have chronic pain and other symptoms, or if you are unable to MELT in the evening, you can MELT in the morning or before or after activities and exercise. What's important is that you make time to learn the method and take time for your self-care so you can have more energy and less pain—and enjoy doing the things you love.

Always Reconnect

Remember the MELT protocol: Reconnect before and after each sequence. At the beginning of each sequence, you will assess to Reconnect to your body's current state. After you MELT, you'll Reconnect again to notice the changes you are making. This allows your Autopilot to reset to a more efficient, balanced state and to recalibrate its connection with your center of gravity.

This is why you will always Reconnect as part of your MELT self-care routine. If you don't, you will miss the opportunity to restore the link between the autonomic nervous system and the connective tissue system, which is how you address the root cause of the four effects of stuck stress. Initially, this is also how you'll know you are MELTing correctly. You can inventory the changes you are making and track your progress.

Use Your Body Sense

Learning how to access your Body Sense can take practice. It is common to be unsure exactly what you feel in your body. This is because you haven't had to access your Body Sense before now. Tapping into your Body Sense is how you get good at using it!

When you're starting out, you may be tempted to touch your body to help you know what you are feeling, but part of helping your Autopilot is learning to use your Body Sense. So if you are not sure what you are feeling, let that be your assessment. Then, once you do the treatment, reassess.

When you're MELTing, take the time to ask yourself, "What am I sensing?" If your answer is, "I feel nothing," it can't hurt to go even slower and use less pressure. When we don't have keen Body Sense, we tend to think we need to press harder so we feel more. If you feel tenderness or sensitivity, approach the area gently and remember to "get in and get out"—you don't want to overstay your welcome.

Don't Inflict Pain

In addition to using your Body Sense to notice positive changes as you MELT, you also need to pay attention to pain. No part of MELT should ever hurt—not during *or* after a MELT session. In fact, pain acts as a barometer: if you are overdoing it during any

MELT session, one of the ways your body will tell you this is with pain. An increase in pain is your signal that you may be moving too fast or applying too much pressure, especially in the beginning. So slow down and ease up. If your pain increases after you MELT, that's also a sign that you need to MELT for less time with less compression (or that your pain was caused by something completely unrelated to MELT).

Indirect Before Direct

Each MELT sequence creates changes directly where you are working. However, what's profound is that you may experience changes far away from where you are MELTing. I know the tendency is to want to go right to where you have pain, but when you have pain, I always recommend that you MELT other parts of your body first. This indirectly rehydrates the troubled area without overstressing the nervous system. This is what I call the Indirect Before Direct approach, which is without a doubt the most effective way to eliminate pain.

Less Is More

No matter how good you get at MELT, ten minutes is the maximum time you should have the roller compressing any mass at a time. Even if it "feels so good," you've only got ten minutes. (If you haven't finished a move or a sequence, you can always come off the roller, reassess, then get back on to finish up.) The connective tissue and nervous systems are quick to respond and adapt when you get in and get out. Take too long, and it's as if they ignore your intervention.

> **Body Changes:** Here are some of the changes you may notice when you add MELT to your routine:
>
> • You sleep better.
> • You have improved body ease.
> • Your daily energy and mood improve.
> • You have better balance and flexibility.

Track Your Results

As you assess and reassess, you'll start to notice that your body has some common imbalances and that MELT helps you address them. Pay attention to what you feel—and how you feel after you MELT. Over time, you'll likely notice that your self-treatment is making some larger changes in your body than just pain relief. You might find it empowering to track these changes.

You may have a list of things you'd like to improve. Perhaps you have neck pain or don't sleep through the night. Maybe you have digestive trouble or weight issues. Take a moment and think about any changes you'd like to make. Keep track of these as you move forward with MELT.

If you aren't seeing any immediate changes, drink more water and keep MELTing. With patience and persistence, you should start to notice changes within two weeks.

▶ Drink Water!

For the best and most lasting results, it's important to drink water before and immediately after you MELT. At least eight ounces of water before and after you MELT should do it. MELT pulls a lot of fluid into your tissues, so it's vital that you hydrate your body if you want to rehydrate your connective tissue.

You can support the efficiency of your body by drinking small amounts of water consistently throughout the day. One quick way to calculate how much water you should drink is to take your body weight in pounds and divide it in half to get the number of ounces you should drink. For example, a 160-pound man or woman should drink eighty ounces of water per day. This is the minimum amount of water your body needs to restore you to a healthier, pain-free state. Also, eat water-filled, nutritious foods, such as fruits and vegetables. Try to stay away from sugary and processed foods, as they increase inflammation and stress in your body. You might find it helpful to keep a food and activity journal to identify what does and doesn't agree with your body.

I recommend that you not drink a lot of water while you're eating. Instead, drink water an hour before and after you eat a meal. When you're drinking small amounts of water consistently, you might find that what you thought were hunger pains between meals were just your body asking for more water.

▶ Special Circumstances

If you are currently under a doctor's care, you can still MELT with permission from your physician. MELT is an ideal complement to physical therapy and rehabilitation. Regardless of your circumstances, your first week will begin with the Hand and Foot Treatment and Rebalance Sequence in this chapter. However, there are special self-treatment plans for your second week and beyond, including customized guidelines, modifications, and maps for the following circumstances:

- Pain due to trauma, injury, or surgery
- Diagnosed systemic conditions, disorders, and diseases
- Pregnancy and postpartum

For a more detailed list of special circumstances and the customized approaches associated with them, see Chapter 14, "MELT as Complementary Self-Care."

▶ Ready, Set, MELT!

To get started, try the following Rebalance Sequence and the Hand and/or Foot Treatment in the evening, up to an hour before bedtime. It's best to try the sequences separately at first, and then you can combine them as you become more familiar with them. Do each sequence at least two to three times your first week. Remember, MELT is so gentle that you can do these sequences every day. This is the foundation of all MELT self-treatment plans.

Rebalance Sequence

This sequence is most effective when done in a quiet area so you are able to focus inward.

Rest Assess	**3-D Breath Breakdown**
Gentle Rocking	**3-D Breath**
Pelvic Tuck and Tilt	**Rest Reassess**

Rest Assess

▶ *Lie on the floor, with your arms and legs straight and relaxed, palms face up.*

▶ *Take a focused breath and allow your body to relax into the floor. Close your eyes and take a moment to sense what you feel. Don't adjust or touch your body—just take notice.*

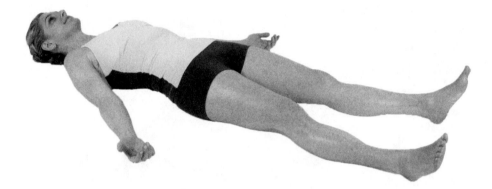

Remember, there are three areas stuck stress loves to live: the shoulder girdle, the diaphragm, and the pelvis. Using Body Sense, scan your body and notice what you feel.

▶ *Assess stuck stress in your shoulder girdle. Does your upper body feel heaviest on your shoulder girdle rather than the middle of your rib cage? Is your head tilting back or resting off center? Do your arms feel out of balance?*

▶ *Turn your head left and right. Do you feel pain or limited range?*

▶ *Assess stuck stress in your diaphragm. Does your low back curve feel more like a mid-back curve?*

▶ *Take a focused breath. Do you sense any restriction as you inhale?*

▶ *Assess stuck stress in your pelvis. Does your pelvis feel more weighted on the tailbone than on your butt cheeks? Do the backs of your thighs feel unevenly weighted or entirely off the floor? Do your feet point out toward the sides of the room or up to the ceiling?*

▶ *Assess your Autopilot. Imagine dividing yourself into right and left sides. Does one entire side of your body feel more weighted to the floor, or does one leg feel longer than the other?*

Gentle Rocking

▶ *Sit next to the bottom of the roller and lean away from it. Put your hands behind you, and then shift your pelvis onto the roller.*

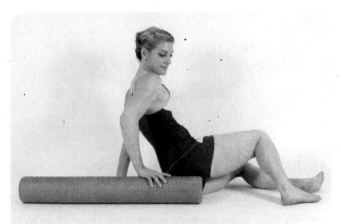

▶ *Using your hands for support, slowly roll yourself down along the length of the roller.*

If you need additional support, place towels, pillows, or bolsters on either side of the roller.

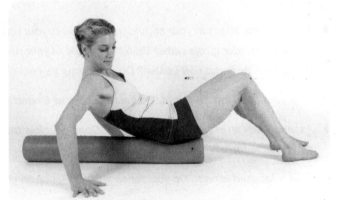

- *Touch the top of your head to make sure it is fully supported by the roller. Make sure your pelvis is on the roller and your feet are flat on the floor, approximately hip-width apart.*

- *Place your forearms on the floor and take a breath.*

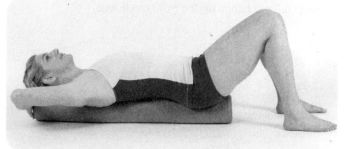

- *Allow your head, chest, and pelvis to slowly tip toward the floor on one side. Then come back through the center and slowly tip toward the other side. You want to get a sense of gently falling and catching yourself with your forearm, while keeping the back of your head, your spine, and the center of your pelvis aligned and heavy on the roller at all times. Continue to gently rock from side to side for about 30 seconds.*

- *Remember, every time you get on the roller, you'll start by gently rocking your body from side to side. This allows your Autopilot to adapt to the pressure on your spine, and it heightens the Autopilot's connection to your center of gravity as you challenge your balance on the unstable surface of the roller. This move is small and subtle when done correctly.*

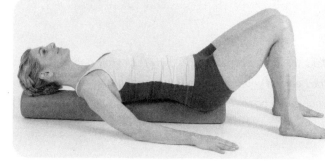

- *Notice what you feel: Do you tip your body weight more easily to one side than to the other?*

- *Return to the center.*

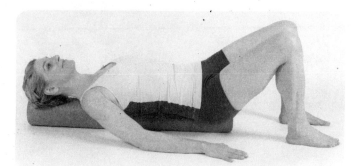

Pelvic Tuck and Tilt

▶ *Place your hands on your pelvis, with your fingertips on the pubic bone and the heels of your hands on the front hip bones.*

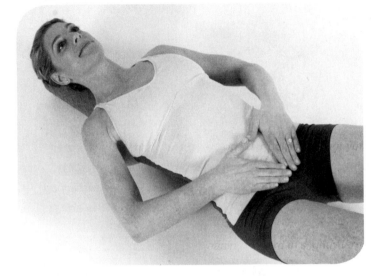

▶ *Take a focused breath and slowly tuck your pelvis. When you tuck your pelvis, the heels of your hands get heavy, your low back travels toward the roller, and your pubic bone rises. Keep your ribs stable and your foot pressure constant.*

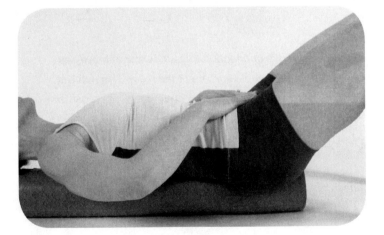

▶ Next, keep your ribs heavy and slowly tilt your pelvis. When you tilt your pelvis, your fingertips get heavy, your pubic bone sinks, and your low back travels away from the roller. Keep your ribs stable as your low back lifts slightly.

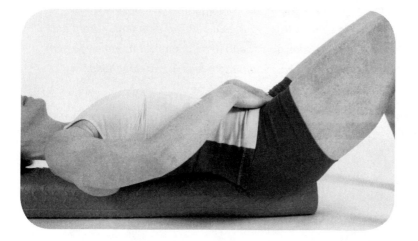

▶ Repeat the tuck and tilt 5–6 times, moving slowly. Keep your feet light on the floor and your ribs relaxed and still.

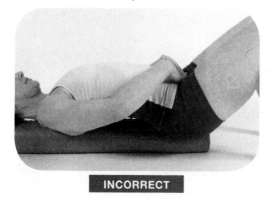

INCORRECT

Make sure you aren't squeezing your butt cheeks or lifting your hips as you tuck and tilt. Don't push into your feet to tuck or let your ribs lift away from the roller when you tilt. The size of the movement is very small and isolated when you perform this move correctly.

Remember, if you notice that your body is rocking slightly left and right, let it happen. This is a good indication that your Autopilot is reconnecting to your center of gravity.

3-D Breath Breakdown

▶ *Place one hand on your chest and the other on your belly.*

▶ *Take 3–4 breaths into the area between the front and the back of your body, allowing the diaphragm to expand from your center in two directions—front and back—as you inhale. These breaths don't need to be the fullest breaths you can take. Instead, focus on expanding your diaphragm in only two directions.*

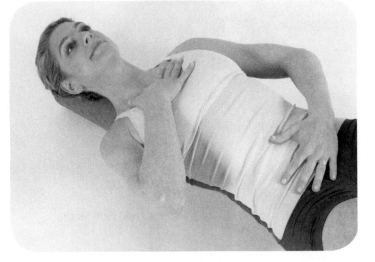

▶ *Place your hands on the widest part of your rib cage, below your armpits. Take 3–4 breaths, allowing the diaphragm to expand between your hands. Find the width of your breath. See if you can sense your hands and ribs moving apart on the inhale. The movement is subtle.*

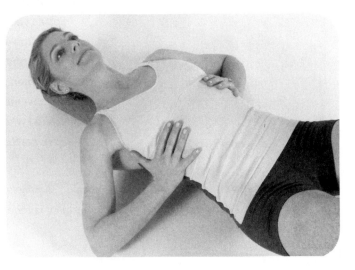

▶ *Place one hand on your collarbones, at the base of the throat, and the other on your pubic bone, at the base of the belly. Take 3–4 focused breaths between them, sending your breath all the way down to your pelvis and all the way up to the top of your lungs at the same time.*

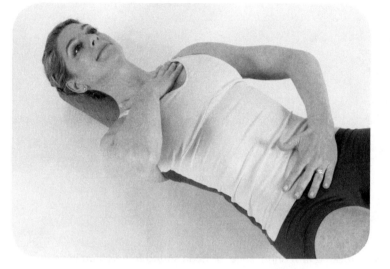

▶ *Notice if your body shifts or the roller rocks a little during any of these directional breaths. This is a good indication that your Autopilot is resetting and acquiring its GPS signal to your center of gravity.*

3-D Breath

▶ *Place both hands on your belly and take a focused breath into all six sides of your torso, expanding three-dimensionally. Notice how your belly expands into your hands on the inhale, and away from them naturally on your exhale. Try this 2–3 times.*

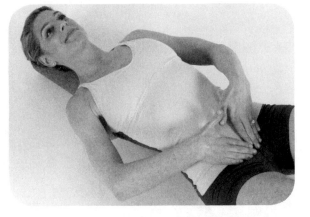

▶ *On your next exhale, make a firm* shhh, seee, *or* haaa *sound to heighten your ability to sense the reflexive action in your deep abdomen. Try all three sounds and sense the cylindrical contraction that subtly squeezes your spine, pelvic floor, and organs from all sides as you force the exhale.*

▶ *Pick the sound that allows you to sense this inward contraction or hugging sensation in your belly best, and use that sound a few more times.*

▶ *Then, without using the sound or forcing an exhale, see if you can use your Body Sense to feel and follow that same reflexive action, starting with your natural exhale and then consciously connecting to the more subtle sensation of engagement.*

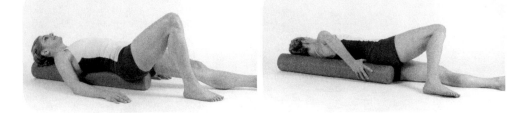

▶ *Try this 2–3 times. This is what we call finding your core. You will be asked to find your core in other moves, so remember this sensation.*

▶ *Slowly come off the roller by placing your hands on the floor, straightening out one leg, and sliding off that side—first with your pelvis, then your ribs and head.*

Rest Reassess

▶ *Lie on the floor with your arms and legs straight and relaxed, palms face up, as you did before. Breathe and allow your body to relax into the floor. Close your eyes and take a moment to reassess.*

▶ *Remember how your body felt when you did your Rest Assess. Use your Body Sense to notice if you've helped eliminate any accumulated stress.*

▶ *Turn your head from left to right. Do you have more range of motion? Is there less pain or stiffness as you turn your head?*

▶ *If you felt like your upper body was heaviest on your shoulder girdle, do you feel more weight in the middle of your rib cage?*

▶ *Do you feel like your low back curve is closer to your pelvis?*

▶ *If you felt like your pelvis was more weighted on the tailbone than on your butt cheeks, notice if you've made any changes there. And what about your thighs: Do they feel heavier and more evenly weighted?*

▶ *Here's the most important thing: Divide yourself into right and left sides. Do you feel more even and balanced from side to side? If so, you've improved your Autopilot's connection to your center of gravity, so it can function more efficiently.*

▶ *Take a breath. Do you feel like you can breathe more easily or more fully?*

▶ *If you sense any of these changes, your body is Rebalancing.*

Soft Ball Foot Treatment

Body Scan Assess

Autopilot Assess

Position Point Pressing

Glide

Shear

Rinse

Friction

Body Scan Reassess

Final Body Scan Reassess

Autopilot Reassess

Body Scan Assess

▶ *Stand with your feet side by side, hip-width apart (approximately 6 inches). Close your eyes and use your Body Sense to notice your feet. Does it feel like you have more weight on your left or right side? Are you sensing that your weight is concentrated on a particular region of your feet?*

▶ *Use your Body Sense to scan up your legs. Notice the joints of your ankles, knees, and hips. Notice your muscles. Are your legs tense? Are your thigh and butt muscles engaged? See if you can relax these muscles and still remain standing comfortably. If so, you are working too hard to simply stand up.*

Autopilot Assess

▶ *Keep your eyes closed and legs relaxed. Lift all ten toes off the floor and take 3 breaths.*

▶ *On the final exhale, set your toes down. Notice if you feel yourself drift forward. That drift is a sign that your Autopilot is having trouble finding your center of gravity.*

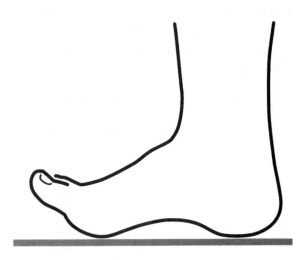

- *Try the same assessment with your eyes open and notice how much less you drift when you can rely on your sense of sight to remain balanced.*

- *After assessing, begin by performing all the techniques on one foot. Then switch to the other foot and do all the techniques.*

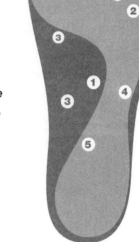

Position Point Pressing

- *Stand up straight with your feet hip-width apart. Place the soft ball on the floor in front of you and step onto it so the ball aligns with position point 1.*

- *Put your feet side by side and gently shift some of your body weight onto the ball to create tolerable pressure. Then shift some of your weight off the ball.*

- *Repeat this shifting 2–3 times to ease into tolerable compression while you take focused breaths.*

- *Step backward with the opposite foot and shift your weight to that foot.*

- *Place the ball under position point 2, directly under the big toe knuckle. Gently rock forward to apply tolerable compression to that point.*

- *Step on your back foot to decompress the ball as you move to the next knuckle. Continue this rocking motion as you compress and decompress each point at the front of the foot, and then move on to position points 3, 4, and 5.*

Glide

- *Place the ball on point 5, right in front of the heel. The ball of your foot and your toes are on the floor. Your heel is off the ground.*

- *Keeping the front of your foot on the floor, slowly move the ball from side to side in front of the heel.*

- *Continue Gliding the ball from side to side as you work your way to the back of the heel and then back to point 5.*

Shear

- *With the ball on point 5, use a slightly heavier compression to wiggle your foot left to right. The ball should barely move.*

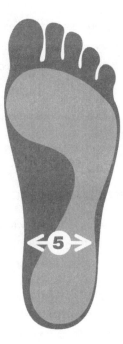

Rinse

- *Place the ball on point 2, directly under the big toe knuckle.*

- *Keeping your heel on the floor, gently press the ball with consistent pressure across the knuckles, toward the outside of the foot. Lift your foot to return to the starting point and repeat 2 more times.*

Remember, you only Rinse in one direction.

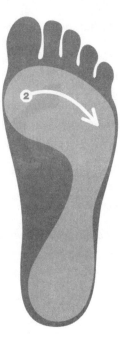

- *Place the ball on point 2 again, directly under the big toe knuckle. Press the ball toward your heel in a continuous motion with tolerable, consistent pressure. For the greatest result, begin your Rinse with your foot slightly behind you so you can easily create a smooth toe-to-heel Rinse.*

- *Lift your foot, place the ball under the next knuckle, and Rinse.*

- *Repeat for all five knuckles.*

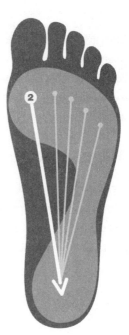

Friction

- *Using light, quick, random movements, rub your foot and toes over the ball in a scribble-like motion.*

Body Scan Reassess

- *Close your eyes and use your Body Sense to notice the side of the body you just self-treated. Notice your foot. Does it feel different than the other foot?*

- *Notice the joints of your leg. You may find that you don't sense the leg as separate parts anymore, and instead your leg feels more cohesive. Notice if you feel more grounded. If you have room, take a few steps and notice the difference between your left and right sides.*

Now repeat all of the techniques on the other foot.

Final Body Scan Reassess

▶ *Close your eyes and use your Body Sense to feel your feet on the floor. Notice your joints. Do your legs feel more cohesive on both sides now? Do you feel more evenly grounded?*

Autopilot Reassess

▶ *Stand with your eyes closed and raise your toes again. When you set your toes back down, do you drift less than you did before? The Soft Ball Foot Treatment improves your Autopilot's connection to your body's center of gravity.*

Soft Ball Hand Treatment

Wrist Assess	Rinse
Grip Assess	Finger Rinse
Finger Compression	Friction
Position Point Pressing	Wrist Reassess
Glide	Grip Reassess
Shear	

Wrist Assess

▶ *Bring your elbows and wrists together.*

▶ *Open your hands so that your palms face the ceiling. Ideally, your hands should look like the letter* T. *If your hands look more like a* Y *or you notice that your pinky finger bends, that's a sign that there's dehydration and unnecessary tension running from your hands all the way to your neck and shoulders, which may be contributing to pain, stiffness, and poor posture.*

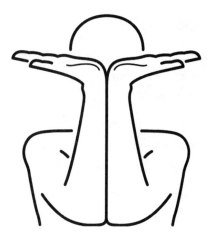

Grip Assess

▶ *Place a soft ball in one hand and squeeze it 3–4 times as firmly as you can.*

▶ *Then place the ball in the other hand and notice whether your grip feels equal in strength or if you have a stronger grip in one hand than in the other. Remember how this feels.*

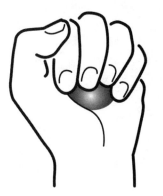

Finger Compression

▶ *Hold the ball in the palm of one hand. Place the pad of your index finger of that hand on top of the ball. If you have trouble keeping the ball in place, you can use your other hand to help hold it.*

▶ *Press down on the ball with the pad of your index finger.*

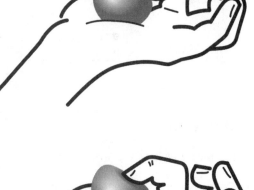

▶ *Then decompress the ball and flex your index finger so your fingertip is touching the ball. Again, compress the ball with mild pressure.*

▶ *Alternate between pressing the tip and the pad of your index finger against the ball 4 times each.*

▶ *Move the ball over a bit in your palm and place your middle finger on top of the ball.*

▶ *Repeat the pattern of flexion and extension 4 times per finger, including your thumb.*

▶ *Switch hands and repeat.*

If you find that you can't make your fingers move one at a time, put two fingers on the ball and see if that's any better. You can even use your other hand to help move the joints when you first try this technique.

Position Point Pressing

▶ *Place the ball on a table or other flat, hard surface. Press your hand into the soft ball at each of the points on the diagram, starting with point 1. Create a tolerable amount of pressure and take a focused breath. You can use your other hand to create gentle compression.*

▶ *Then compress points 2 through 5, starting under your index finger. At each point, take a focused breath before lifting your hand and moving to the next point. Ease off the pressure if you feel a strong sensation or pain. This is a very powerful technique, so take your time.*

▶ *Once you've pressed into each point, repeat on the other hand.*

Glide

▶ *On your right hand, with your palm down, Glide the soft ball from point 3 across the base of the palm to point 5 and return to point 3 with consistent pressure. Keep the tip of your middle finger on the table or floor as you create the Glide. Continue back and forth as you take 3–4 focused breaths.*

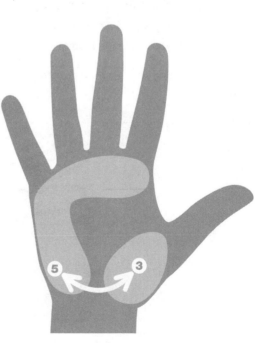

Shear

▶ *Place the soft ball under point 3, the thumb pad, on your right hand and create small circles as you take 3–4 focused breaths. Move slowly and take your time with Shearing the thumb pad, as this area often carries a lot of stuck stress.*

▶ *Repeat the Glide and Shear on the left hand.*

Rinse

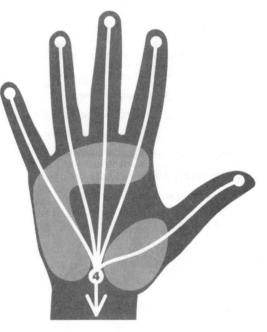

▶ *Starting at the tip of one finger on your right hand, slowly press the soft ball down the finger, across point 4, and over your wrist.*

▶ *Repeat, starting at the tip of each of the other fingers.*

▶ *Switch hands and repeat.*

▶ *Next, start at the fingertip and slowly press the soft ball through your wrist and up your forearm in a continuous motion until you reach the elbow.*

▶ *Repeat, starting from each of the other fingers.*

▶ *Switch hands and repeat.*

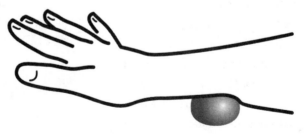

Finger Rinse

▶ *Place your left hand flat on the floor or a table. Use the right hand to rub the soft ball over the top of and in between each finger of the left hand in one direction, from the knuckle to the nail. (This also stimulates point 4 on the top hand, rehydrating the tissues of the wrist, reducing inflammation, and relieving wrist pain.)*

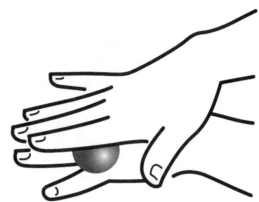

▶ *Repeat on the other hand.*

Friction

▶ *Using light, quick, random movements, rub one hand over the soft ball in a scribble-like motion. Be sure to include your fingers and wrist.*

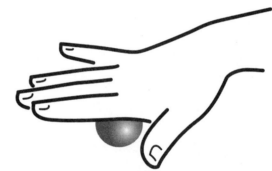

▶ *Repeat on the other hand.*

Wrist Reassess

As you know by now, assessing yourself is crucial.

▶ *Bring your elbows and wrists together. Open your hands so that your palms face the ceiling. Do you feel a change in the flexibility of your wrists? Do you feel less tension in your arms? Do your fingers extend more fully?*

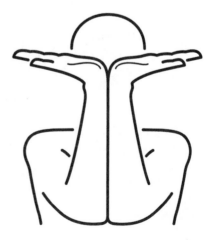

Grip Reassess

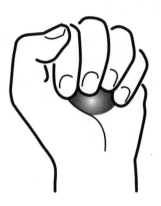

▶ *Remember what your grip strength felt like when you began and repeat the Grip Assess. Place a soft ball in one hand and squeeze it 3–4 times as firmly as you can. Repeat with the other hand. Can you now create a more powerful grip with less effort? Does your grip feel more equal from left to right?*

11

Rehydrate the Upper and Lower Body

Now that you have Reconnected to your Autopilot, helped it acquire its GPS signal to your center of gravity, and Rebalanced your NeuroCore, it's time to get a handle on the stuck stress in your connective tissue and sense what it feels like to make changes in your own body.

You have learned about the Rehydrate techniques of Gliding, Shearing, Rinsing, and Two-Directional Length, and you practiced these techniques on your calf and the back of your leg. Now you can apply these techniques to the masses of your body, where so much stuck stress is wreaking havoc on your primary spaces.

When you Glide, Shear, and Rinse the larger masses of your upper and lower body, you get the tensional energy back into a cohesive, whole-body flow. Rehydrating these masses improves spinal stability and helps restore the mobility and stability of joints throughout the body, including your knees, shoulders, neck, and hips. Pain in all of these joints can be reduced and even eliminated with the Rehydrate techniques.

With MELT Rehydrate techniques, your repetitive habits of sitting, standing, or playing sports won't create chronic pain and stuck stress. Your daily activities will no longer cause unnecessary stiffness or joint compression. Try the following Rehydrate sequences in the evening, up to an hour before bedtime. Try the Lower Body Compression and Length Sequences one evening and the Upper Body Compression and Length Sequences on another, at least two times a week. Continue to do your Rebalance Sequence and the Hand and/or Foot Treatment three times a week, either together with one of these sequences or separately. Pay attention to the length of time you are on the roller as you learn these techniques. Remember, ten minutes is the maximum amount of time you should compress any area of your body on the roller. You can come off the roller at any time, reassess, and go back to the move or sequence.

Remember to drink a glass of water before and after every MELT session. It's part of the treatment and will help you get the most out of MELT.

Lower Body Compression Sequence

Rest Assess

Back Thigh Shear

Calf Glide and Shear

Inner Thigh Glide and Shear

Calf Rinse

Inner and Back Thigh Rinse

Rest Reassess

Rest Assess

▶ *Lie on the floor with your arms and legs straight and relaxed, palms face up. Take a breath and allow your body to relax into the floor.*

▶ *Remember, if all your upper back weight is on your shoulder blades, if your mid-back is arched off the floor, if your tailbone is more weighted than your butt cheeks, or if the backs of your thighs feel off the floor on one or both sides, you have identified stuck stress in your body.*

▶ *Close your eyes and, using your Body Sense, notice what you feel.*

▶ *Turn your head left and right. Do you feel pain or limited range?*

▶ Bring your attention to the curve of your low back. Using your navel as a reference point, does your back feel lifted off the floor from the navel to the shoulder blades? Take note of what you feel.

▶ Notice your pelvis. Ideally, you feel two butt cheeks evenly weighted on the floor. Notice if you sense your tailbone on the floor instead of your butt cheeks or if one side of your pelvis feels more weighted than the other.

▶ Bring your attention to your thighs. Ideally they touch the floor evenly on both sides. How much of your thighs do you feel on the floor? Does one thigh feel heavier to the floor than the other? You may not feel your thighs touching the floor at all—just make a note of what you feel.

▶ Notice whether you feel a space behind both of your knees and whether the calves weight evenly. The ankles are a space, and the heels rest on the floor. Ideally, you're resting on the outer third of your heels, with your toes pointing toward where the walls meet the ceiling.

▶ Notice your legs from hip to heel. Does the right or the left leg feel heavier or longer, or do they feel even?

▶ Finally, take a full breath and notice what areas of your torso move when your lungs fill with air. Does your belly move? Ribs? Both? Just sense what moves and what doesn't.

▶ Take note of what you feel so you can compare after you complete the Lower Body Compression Sequence.

Back Thigh Shear

▶ *Lie on your back with your knees bent. Place the roller underneath the backs of your thighs, just below the crease of your buttocks.*

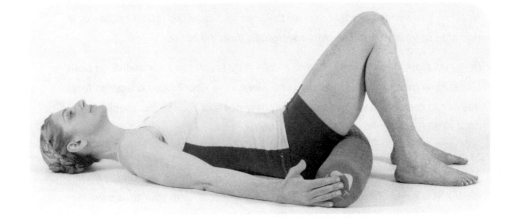

▶ *Let your upper body relax on the floor as you straighten your legs. Relax your legs and keep them heavy on the roller.*

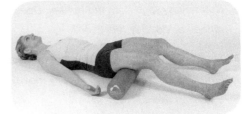

▶ *Keep your feet close to the floor as you Shear the backs of your thighs by dragging your legs together and apart while maintaining consistent pressure on top of the roller. Turn your legs inward as you draw your legs together and outward as you draw them apart. Think of twisting your flesh around the thigh bone rather than rubbing your thighs on the roller as you repeat this movement 4–5 times.*

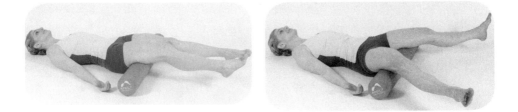

> *Try it one leg at a time: Bend one leg and relax it on the roller, and then drag and twist the other leg in and out. Keep the compression tolerable and consistent as you drag your leg in and out 4–5 times.*

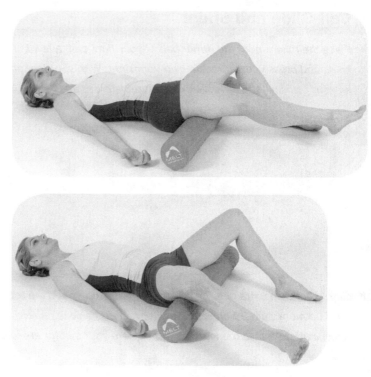

> *Repeat with the other thigh 4–5 times.*

> *Return your legs to the center, pause for 2 focused breaths, and allow your upper thighs to sink further into the roller.*

> *Move the roller down to the middle of your thighs (where cellulite often appears) and repeat the Shear. You can Shear both legs at the same time or just one leg at a time. Repeat this twisting action 4–5 times, and then return your legs to the center, pause, and take a focused breath.*

> *Move the roller down once more to the area just above your knees.*

> *Repeat Shearing both legs together or one leg at a time, 4–5 times.*

> *When you are done, pause, wait, and take a focused breath.*

Calf Glide and Shear

▶ *Place the roller under the upper half of your right calf, a few inches below your knee, and cross your left ankle over your right. With your feet and legs relaxed, let your calf sink into the roller with tolerable pressure.*

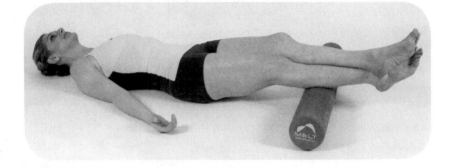

▶ *Slowly bend and straighten your knee 4–5 times to move the roller back and forth no more than 2 inches. Keep your feet and ankles relaxed and maintain a consistent, tolerable pressure as you explore your calf for areas of stuck stress.*

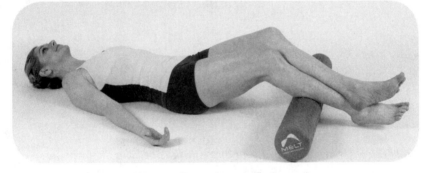

▶ *Rotate your calf outward and repeat the small back-and-forth Gliding motion 3–4 times.*

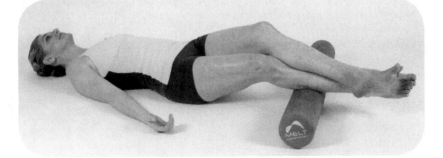

- *Then rotate your calf inward and Glide 3–4 times.*

- *Use your Body Sense to notice which of the three areas feels more tender.*

- *Return to that area and continue to Glide, making the movement smaller and smaller for 2–3 breaths.*

- *Now pause, maintain tolerable pressure, and indirectly Shear by flexing and pointing your right ankle 3–4 times and then making circles with your ankle 3–4 times in each direction.*

- *Relax your ankle and create a direct Shear by turning your right leg in and out in a small, controlled movement, 1–2 inches, 4–5 times. The roller remains stationary.*

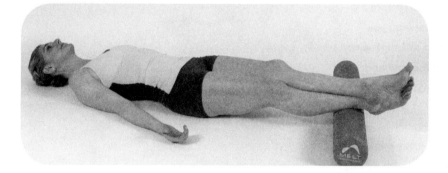

- *Maintain compression of your calf on the roller, and gently shift your leg slightly left to right, like you're scratching the calf against the roller. This is called cross friction.*

  If you feel any pain, reduce the pressure by uncrossing your legs.

- *Pause, wait, and take 2 focused breaths while you let the calf sink further into the roller.*

- *Move the roller down to the lower half of your right calf, a few inches above your ankle. Repeat the same Glide and Shear techniques in this region.*

- *Switch legs and repeat the entire sequence on the other calf.*

Inner Thigh Glide and Shear

▶ *Lie on your right side and place the roller in front of you. Place your left inner thigh on top of the roller, just above your knee.*

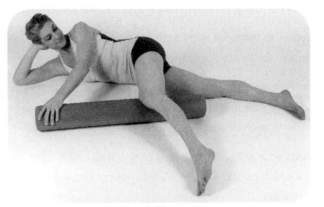

▶ *Push the top end of the roller away from you. The roller will angle away from your upper body, like you're making the letter V. Let your head rest on your lower arm or use a pillow for more neck support. Place your left hand on the floor.*

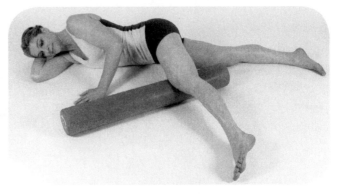

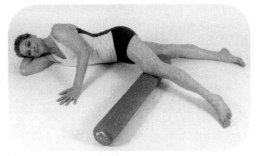

If you are unable to elevate the leg as shown, angle the top of the roller farther away from your upper body.

▶ *Begin to Glide by allowing your body to fall slightly forward. Then, using your left arm, push your body back so the roller moves 1–2 inches up and down your lower inner thigh, just above your knee, 4–5 times.*

- Then turn your leg inward so your toes point down to the floor and Glide 4–5 times. When you find an area of stuck stress, make your Glide smaller and smaller on this area and then edge up against it and pause.

- Take a focused breath and begin an indirect Shear by slowly bending and straightening your knee 3 times. Keep the lower leg relaxed and the pressure on the roller consistent.

- Create a direct Shear by rotating the bent leg, so your foot goes up and then down to the floor 3 times.

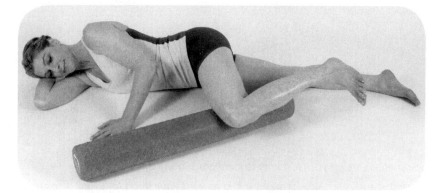

- Let your foot relax on the floor and try cross friction, by pushing into your foot to twist the flesh of your thigh against the roller in a slow scratching motion 3–4 times.

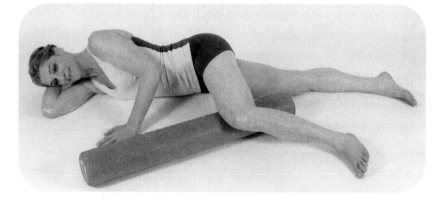

This area is often very tender when you first begin MELTing, so don't be surprised if it feels sensitive. Remember, use tolerable pressure. If it is painful, lighten up your pressure on the roller.

▶ Straighten your knee, and with a relaxed leg, pause and take 2 focused breaths while you let your thigh compress and sink further into the roller.

▶ Move the roller to the middle of your thigh and reset your body position. Rest your head on your right arm. Place your left hand on the floor.

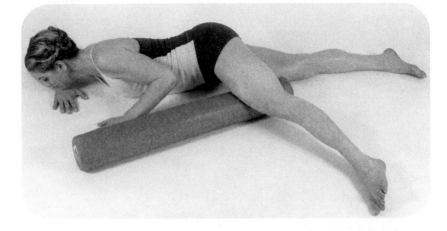

▶ Begin Gliding again, using your left arm to push your body back and fall forward. Breathe and relax as you explore this area of your thigh for stuck stress by turning your thigh slightly inward and outward as you Glide 4–5 times.

When you find an area of stuck stress, Glide in smaller movements, and pause right next to this tender spot to Shear.

▶ Maintain tolerable pressure and repeat your indirect Shear by bending and straightening your knee 3 times. Keeping your knee bent, lift and lower the foot for the direct Shear. You can also "scratch" the inner thigh up and down the roller, twisting the flesh to create cross friction.

▶ Straighten your knee, relax your leg, and allow the weight of your leg to rest on top of the roller as you take 2 focused breaths.

▶ Repeat this sequence one more time, finding another spot on the upper third of your inner thigh.

▶ Repeat the entire sequence on your right inner thigh.

Calf Rinse

▶ *Sit on the floor and place your arms behind you for support. With your right knee bent, rotate your right leg inward and place your inner ankle on the roller. Your foot is relaxed, and your big toe is close to the floor.*

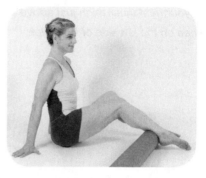

▶ *Lean forward and slowly straighten your right leg to allow the roller to move up your inner calf with consistent, light pressure. It's okay if the roller doesn't travel all the way up your calf.*

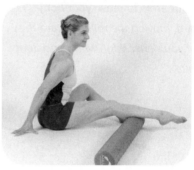

▶ *Rotate your leg so the back of your leg is on the roller.*

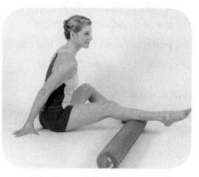

▶ *Lean back and slowly bend your knee to allow the roller to move down the back of your calf with consistent, light pressure. Stop before your ankle and repeat the Rinse 3–4 times.*

▶ *Repeat on the other leg.*

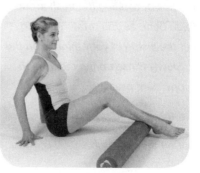

REHYDRATE THE UPPER AND LOWER BODY

Inner and Back Thigh Rinse

▶ *Place your right inner thigh just above the knee on the left side of the roller.*

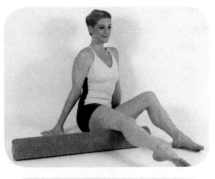

▶ *Use your arms to move your body forward, moving the roller toward the top of your inner thigh with consistent pressure.*

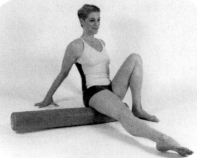

▶ *When you reach the top, think of twisting the flesh around the thigh bone as you rotate your leg so the back of your upper thigh is on the roller.*

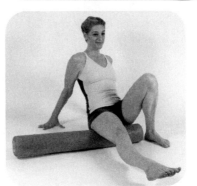

▶ *Use your arms to move your body backward, moving the roller down your thigh with consistent pressure. Stop right above your knee.*

▶ *Again think of twisting the flesh around the thigh bone as you rotate your leg so that the inside of your thigh is on the roller. Slowly Rinse up the inner thigh with consistent pressure.*

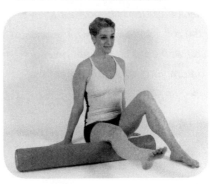

▶ *Repeat this Rinsing pass 3–4 times.*

▶ *Repeat on the left thigh.*

Rest Reassess

▶ *Lie on the floor with your arms and legs straight and relaxed, palms face up. Breathe and allow your body to relax into the floor. Close your eyes and take a moment to reassess.*

▶ *Remember the four common imbalances. Did you make changes? Do your ribs feel more weighted to the floor? Is your low back curve more relaxed and closer to your pelvis? Is your pelvis more weighted on your butt cheeks than on your tailbone? Have the backs of your thighs settled to the floor?*

▶ *Turn your head from left to right. Do you have more range of motion? Is there less pain or stiffness as you turn your head?*

▶ *Bring your attention to your pelvis. If during your first Rest Assess your tailbone was the most noticeable part of your pelvis on the floor, notice if you now sense your butt cheeks more.*

▶ *Notice your legs. Are the backs of your thighs more settled on the floor? Do the right and left sides feel more even?*

▶ *Finally, take a full breath and notice if you sense greater movement. Is it easier to take a deep breath?*

▶ *If you sense any of these changes, you have alleviated stuck stress in your body.*

These changes indicate that your body has enough hydration to respond to the self-treatment. You've pulled a lot of fluids into your tissues, so make sure you drink a glass of water within the next twenty minutes.

Lower Body Length Sequence

Rest Assess

SI Joint Shear

Bent Knee Press

Hip to Heel Press

Rest Reassess

Rest Assess

▶ *Lie on the floor with your arms and legs straight and relaxed, palms face up. Take a breath and allow your body to relax into the floor.*

▶ *Remember, if all your upper back weight is on your shoulder blades, if your mid-back is arched off the floor, if your tailbone is more weighted than your butt cheeks, or if the backs of your thighs feel off the floor on one or both sides, you have identified stuck stress in your body.*

▶ *Close your eyes and, using your Body Sense, notice what you feel.*

▶ *Bring your attention to the curve of your low back. Does your back feel lifted off the floor from the navel to the shoulder blades?*

▶ *Notice your pelvis. Notice if you sense your tailbone on the floor instead of your butt cheeks or if one side of your pelvis feels more weighted than the other.*

▶ *Bring your attention to your thighs. How much of your thighs do you feel on the floor? Does one thigh feel heavier to the floor than the other?*

▶ *Finally, take a full breath. Does your belly move? Ribs? Both?*

▶ *Take note of what you feel so you can compare after you complete the Lower Body Length Sequence.*

SI Joint Shear

▶ *Lie on the floor, bend your knees, and put your feet flat on the floor, hip-width apart.*

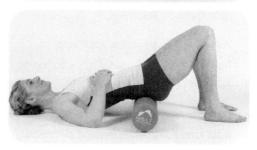

▶ *Place the roller on the floor below your knees. Push your feet into the floor, lift up your hips, and position the roller under the flat part of your pelvis (on the sacrum).*

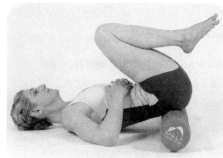

▶ *Draw both knees toward your chest to check if the roller is in the right place. When you bring both knees into your chest, the roller should not slip out or feel like it's under your low back.*

If you have a hard time getting the roller under your pelvis, place a folded yoga mat or towel underneath your head and upper back.

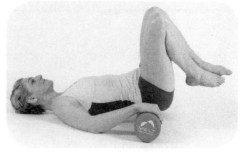

▶ *Keep your knees fully bent, inner thighs together, and relax your lower legs and feet. Keep your core engaged and your ribs relaxed and heavy on the floor.*

Slowly move your knees away from your chest so your knees aim toward the ceiling, but stop before your thighs are fully perpendicular to the roller. This will help keep your low back relaxed.

- *Maintain a consistent pressure and slowly angle your knees slightly right and left between the one and eleven o'clock positions to explore both SI joints.*

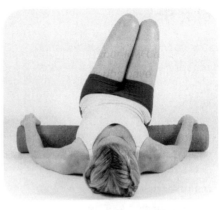

Don't angle your knees too far to either side. Your goal is for your weight to be on the back of the pelvis, not on your hips.

As you move, try not to arch your back or move your ribs. Focus on moving your pelvis and not your ribs by keeping your core engaged.

Pause on the right side and Shear the right SI joint by making small circles with both knees 2–3 times in each direction.

- *Then try circling just the leg you're leaning toward in slightly larger but slower circles.*

- *Also try moving your knees forward and back in a marching motion 2–3 times slowly.*

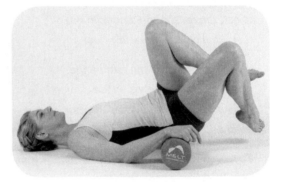

- *Keep your legs tipped to the right side, pause for a moment, maintain the pressure, and take 2 focused breaths.*

- *Return your knees to the center and repeat on the left side.*

Bent Knee Press

▶ *Place the roller under the center of your pelvis. Begin by tucking your pelvis and allowing your ribs to relax and sink into the floor.*

▶ *Engage your core. Lift your right leg up and interlace your hands over the shin or around the back of your thigh.*

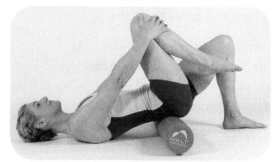

▶ *Keep your left foot firmly on the floor and keep your left knee in line with your hip.*

▶ *Make sure your hips remain level on top of the roller, from left to right. Inhale, and on the exhale, accentuate the tuck of your pelvis and sense the pull on the front of your left thigh. Pause and take a focused breath.*

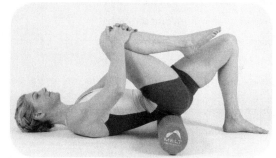

Notice if your left leg swings to the left as you pull your right knee toward your chest. If it does, ease back pressure and reset your left knee so that it points straight ahead.

▶ *Inhale and relax, and then exhale and tuck the pelvis as you draw your right knee toward your torso. Think about your left knee reaching over your left foot in the opposite direction. Take a focused breath. Repeat one more time on this side.*

▶ *Repeat on the other side.*

Hip to Heel Press

▶ *Place your left foot on the floor so your left knee is in line with your hip. Raise your right thigh so your knee points toward the ceiling.*

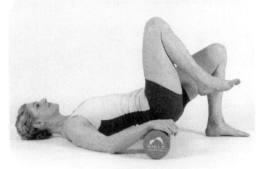

▶ *Straighten your right leg out in front of you and flex your ankle. Keep your pelvis heavy on top of the roller in a slight tilt, and your mid ribs relaxed and weighted to the floor.*

▶ *Keeping your leg straight, slowly bring your flexed right foot toward the ceiling and stop before your knee bends. (Keep the leg straight without locking or hyperextending the knee or creating pain in the knee.)*

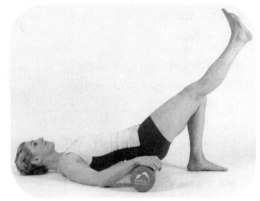

▶ *Even if you are very flexible, don't extend your leg beyond a ninety-degree angle. If your leg is angled toward your nose, you will lose the ability to lengthen the connective tissue on the back of your leg.*

▶ *On an exhale, in two directions, actively flex your ankle and tilt your pelvis, keeping your pelvis weighted to the top of the roller. Take a focused breath as you feel the tensional pull from your heel all the way down to your hip.*

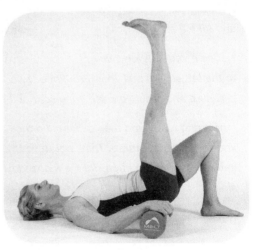

▶ *Inhale and relax the foot. Then exhale and actively flex your foot and allow the pelvis to sink into the roller to find your tilt. Take a focused breath and pause as you accentuate the pull again. Repeat one more time on this side, and then bring your right foot to the floor.*

▶ *Repeat on the other side.*

Rest Reassess

▶ *Lie on the floor with your arms and legs straight and relaxed, palms face up. Breathe and allow your body to relax into the floor. Close your eyes and take a moment to reassess.*

▶ *Remember the four common imbalances. Did you make changes? Do your ribs feel more weighted to the floor? Is your low back curve more relaxed and closer to your pelvis? Is your pelvis more weighted on your butt cheeks than on your tailbone? Have the backs of your thighs settled to the floor?*

▶ *Bring your attention to your pelvis. If during your Rest Assess your tailbone was the most noticeable part of your pelvis on the floor, notice if you now sense your butt cheeks more.*

▶ *Notice your legs. Are the backs of your thighs more settled on the floor?*

▶ *Finally, take a full breath and notice if you sense greater movement. Is it easier to take a deep breath?*

▶ *If you sense any of these changes, your body has returned to a more ideal position.*

▶ Why Rehydrating Your Lower Body Is Important

Although walking seems as easy as putting one foot in front of the other, it's actually very complex. In fact, 80 percent of walking involves balancing on one leg at a time without your conscious awareness. Although your leg muscles move you forward, the fluid communication and stabilizing mechanisms in the connective tissue system are what allow you to stay upright without damaging the many intricate moving parts of your body.

When you have good fluid movement in your connective tissue system, movement of your legs is cohesive and effortless. Communication and vibration can travel clearly and quickly, which is essential to your body's ability to appropriately distribute your weight while making adjustments for changes underfoot, like an uneven surface. Your legs are flexible and stable, and your joints have ease of mobility.

When you have stuck stress in your legs, it interrupts whole-body communication. This leads to joint compression, uncoordinated movement, stiffness, poor balance, muscle tension, inflammation, cartilage breakdown, and pain. Furthermore, stuck stress in your lower body causes imbalance and instability in your NeuroCore, as the legs house the channel for communication from the ground to your pelvis, ribs, and head.

The legs are a long region of the body, with the joints—ankles, knees, and hips—at a great distance from each other. Because of this, good tensional energy in the connective tissue of the legs is all the more vital for stabilization. Without appropriate stability, compensation and joint damage occur. Dehydration in your legs alters the position of your pelvis, ribs, and head and the tensional integrity of your whole body. Over time, spinal instability follows, which leads to low back and neck pain.

What causes stuck stress in your legs? The better question is, What doesn't? Except when you're lying in bed, your legs are supporting the majority of your upper body weight—whether you are moving, standing, or sitting—and this causes dehydration. Basically, living dehydrates your legs, but the greatest offender is sitting. When you sit for long periods of time, you compress your whole backside with your body weight. All the water in your connective tissue "sponge" gets pressed out, and if the connective tissue is not rehydrated, excessive tensional pull becomes a permanent state.

Sitting is the norm in our technology-driven society, and it's having a greater negative impact than you may realize. Studies are finding that sitting for many hours a day causes life-shortening health issues. Sitting hinders cholesterol maintenance. Slowly the enzyme production and utilization that help break down fat drops nearly 90 percent. Meanwhile, good cholesterol drops 20 percent, and insulin synthesis drops nearly 25 percent. Over time your risk of diabetes, heart disease, and obesity increases—even if you live an otherwise healthy lifestyle.

When you sit all day, communication with the NeuroCore significantly decreases and the regulators become chronically imbalanced. The cells within your connective tissue that aid in repair, restoration, and immunity become inflamed and unavailable for healing. Unfortunately, the antidote isn't exercise. Studies show that exercising for an hour a day doesn't counteract the detrimental effects of the eight or more hours of sitting that most Americans do every day.

Cellulite and More

The proof of the physical damage that sitting does to your connective tissue is the lumpy, bumpy, cottage-cheese-like appearance of the skin where you sit. I'm talking about cellulite on people's thighs, of course.

When the backs of your legs are chronically compressed, the tissue becomes dehydrated, and the collagen network in the tissue is damaged. The spongy superficial layers become so dehydrated that fat cells get trapped between the collagen fibers. This further damages the connective tissue and creates a breakdown in the spongy layers, causing the fatty tissue to poke through, leading to the cottage-cheese effect.

Yes, the lumpy appearance of cellulite is caused by dehydrated connective tissue, which is why weight loss alone doesn't solve the issue. Even when you lose weight and reduce body fat, the damaged tissue remains. Rehydrating the backs of your legs with MELT helps! MELT isn't advertised as a cellulite-reduction technique, but maybe it should be. Consider cellulite reduction a wonderful side effect.

Beyond the reduction of cellulite, rehydration of the lower body can quickly yield improvements in flexibility, overall stability, body ease, breathing, and Body Sense. Over time, the agility, balance, and coordination that usually decline as you age can be improved and maintained by rehydrating your legs. If you are an athlete, rehydration of your connective tissue can be your competitive edge, as it improves performance, decreases the risk of injury, and prolongs your career.

Restoring cohesive fluid movement, or tensional energy, to the legs can help you restore low back mobility and spinal stability. Furthermore, rehydrating the legs dramatically improves the tensional energy of the entire connective tissue system, resulting in better alignment, movement, and function of your whole body.

Upper Body Compression Sequence

Rest Assess   Upper Back Rinse

Rib Length Assess   Rib Length Reassess

Upper Back Glide and Shear   Rest Reassess

Shoulder Blade Glide and Shear

Rest Assess

▶ *Lie on the floor with your arms and legs straight and relaxed, palms face up. Take a breath and allow your body to relax into the floor.*

▶ *Remember, if all of your upper back weight is on your shoulder blades, if your mid-back is arched off the floor, if your tailbone is more weighted than your butt cheeks, or if the backs of your thighs feel off the floor on one or both sides, you have identified stuck stress in your body.*

▶ *Close your eyes and, using your Body Sense, notice what you feel.*

▶ *Notice where your head is touching the floor. Is it tilted back? Does it feel off-center?*

▶ *Turn your head left and right. Do you feel pain or limited range?*

▶ *Notice your upper body. Ideally, your upper back is relaxed and resting on your ribs, or mid-back, and not your shoulder blades. Is one shoulder blade more weighted to the floor than the other? Do you feel the edge of either shoulder blade? Are your bottom ribs on or off the floor? Notice your arms. Is the weight of your forearms and upper arms balanced from left to right?*

▶ *Notice the curve of your low back. Does it feel like there's a big curve up toward your shoulder blades, or perhaps there is no curve at all?*

▶ *Finally, take a full breath and notice what areas of your torso expand when your lungs fill with air. Does your belly move? Do your ribs? Both? Just sense what moves and what doesn't.*

▶ *Take note of what you feel so you can compare after you complete the Upper Body Compression Sequence.*

Rib Length Assess

▶ *Rest your shoulder blades on the roller and bend your knees.*

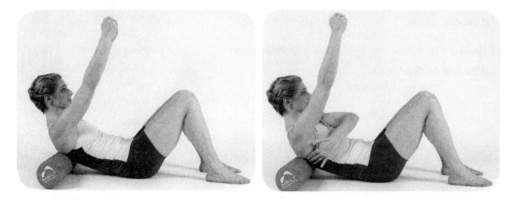

To check your position, lift your arms up and punch toward the ceiling. If you are in the right place on the roller, you should feel your shoulder blades tap the top of the roller. You can also check by reaching one hand around your torso to touch the bottom of the opposite shoulder blade. It should be on the foot side of the roller, not on top of the roller. Adjust if necessary.

▶ *Interlace your hands behind your head and let your neck relax. Tuck your pelvis. As you create the following movement, your core, low back, and neck remain still and stable.*

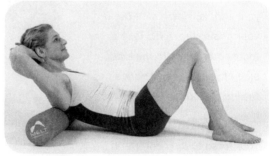

▶ *Breathe in. On the exhale, find your core, allow only your ribs to extend over the roller, and open your breastbone toward the ceiling.*

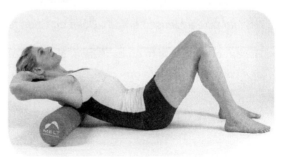

▶ Take 2 focused breaths into your ribs and notice if you feel any stiffness in the front of your chest.

▶ Breathe in, and then on the exhale, curl your ribs forward to the starting position.

▶ Repeat the movement again. Are you able to move your ribs without moving your low back or neck?

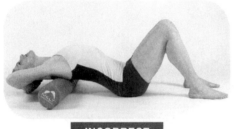

INCORRECT

When you perform this move correctly, the low back and neck curves will remain in the same position as you move your ribs. If you are extending your neck, hanging your head back, or letting your bottom ribs pop up, slow down and make your movement smaller.

▶ Repeat the movement again. This time, from the extended position, breathe in, and on your exhale, slowly side bend your ribs to the right. Take a focused breath into the left side of your ribs and notice the feeling as you breathe.

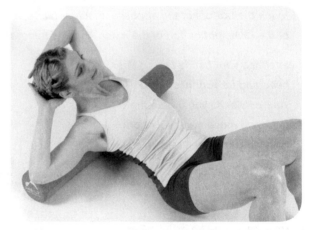

On your next exhale, return your torso to the center and then slowly side bend to the left and take a focused breath. Does one side feel easier to breathe into?

▶ Repeat one more time on each side. Notice if one or both sides feel restricted or if you move more to one side. Then return to the center.

Upper Back Glide and Shear

▶ *Rest your upper back on the roller. Keep your hands behind your head for support and point your elbows toward the ceiling. Engage your core and lift your hips slightly off the floor to bring the roller to the top of your upper back. Keep your pelvis tucked.*

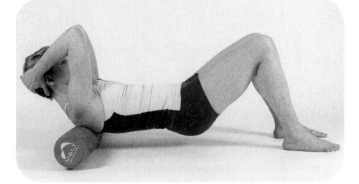

▶ *Keep your back slightly curled forward to maintain the correct position. Focus on keeping your body weight heavy on the top of the roller. Push into your feet to gently Glide the roller up and down 2–3 inches of your upper back 6–8 times. Keep the motion small.*

▶ *Set your hips back down to the floor and curl your ribs forward slightly more. Keep your elbows pointed toward the ceiling. Take a focused breath and Shear by slowly side bending your upper body left and right in small*

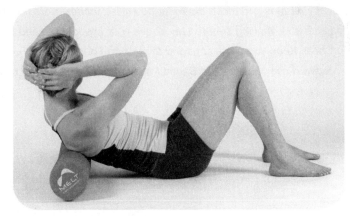

movements 3 times, as if you are scratching an itch on your back. Keep your pressure constant.

▶ *Return to the center, pause, and take a focused breath, letting your spine sink further into the roller.*

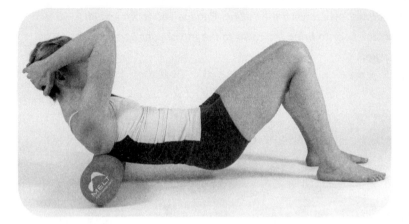

▶ *Lift your hips slightly off the ground and push into your feet to move the roller down your back 1–2 inches, curling your ribs forward. Walk your feet toward your body to maintain good support.*

▶ *Gently Glide up and down the middle of your back, 2–3 inches. Then set your hips on the floor, curl your ribs forward, and Shear by creating a small side bending motion left to right. Pause and take a focused breath.*

▶ *Lift your hips and move the roller down 1–2 inches more, on the bra line or just below, making sure to stay above your lowest ribs, and then Glide and Shear. Keep your core engaged to support your spine and curl your ribs slightly forward as you Glide and Shear. Pause and take a focused breath.*

Shoulder Blade Glide and Shear

▶ *Rest your upper back on the roller with your hands behind your head, knees bent, feet flat on the floor. Keep your core engaged and tip your upper body slightly to the right so the roller is on the bottom of your right shoulder blade, not on your spine. Keep your back curled forward and lift your hips an inch off the floor.*

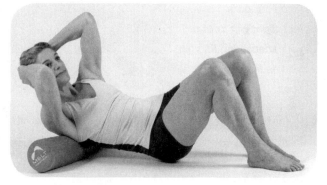

▶ *Using your feet, Glide up and down the bottom and inner edge of your right shoulder blade. If you find a tender spot, make your movement smaller and smaller and edge up against the area of stuck stress but don't land right on it.*

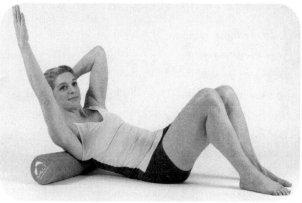

▶ *Set your right buttock to the floor. To Shear, release your right arm from behind your head and slowly create 5–6 small circles or figure 8 movements with your arm in front of your body.*

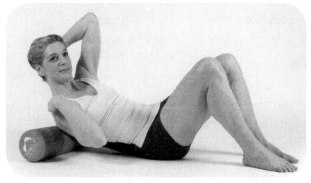

▶ *Bring your hand back behind your head, pause, and take a focused breath, letting your shoulder blade sink further into the roller.*

▶ *Return your body to the center. Then repeat these steps on the other shoulder blade.*

Upper Back Rinse

▶ *Find your core, set your feet slightly in front of your knees, and lift your hips an inch off the floor.*

▶ *Bring your knees over your feet so the roller moves to the upper part of your back. Take a focused breath.*

▶ *On the exhale, engage your core and gently push into your feet to allow the roller to slowly travel down your back with consistent, light pressure. Curl your ribs forward as your legs extend and your hips settle back to the floor.*

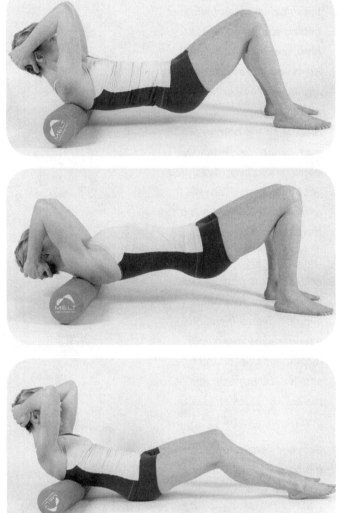

▶ *Reset your feet slightly in front of your knees and then find your core, lift your hips off the floor, and bring your knees over your feet again so the roller moves to your upper back. Pause and take a focused breath.*

▶ *Repeat the Rinse 3–4 times, then reset the roller under your shoulder blades and bend your knees.*

Rib Length Reassess

▶ *With the middle of your shoulder blades resting on top of the roller and your pelvis tucked, breathe in and then, on the exhale, allow only your ribs to extend over the roller again.*

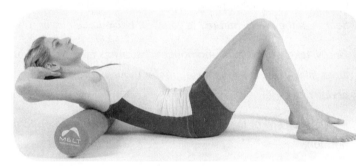

▶ *Notice if you move more freely or sense a greater range of motion in this extended position. Repeat once.*

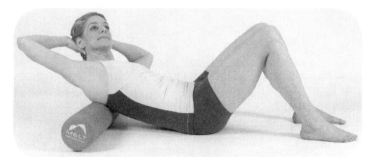

▶ *Maintain this extension and slowly side bend your ribs to the right and take 2–3 focused breaths. Repeat on the left side.*

▶ *Repeat 2 times on each side.*

▶ *Notice if you move more freely or sense a greater range of motion when you side bend than you did before.*

Rest Reassess

▶ *Lie on the floor with your arms and legs straight and relaxed, palms face up. Breathe and allow your body to relax into the floor. Close your eyes and take a moment to reassess.*

▶ *Remember the four common imbalances. Did you make changes? Do your ribs feel more weighted to the floor? Is your low back curve more relaxed and closer to your pelvis? Is your pelvis more weighted on your butt cheeks than on your tailbone? Have the backs of your thighs settled to the floor?*

▶ *Turn your head from left to right. Do you have more range of motion? Is there less pain or stiffness as you turn your head?*

▶ *Notice whether your upper body is more relaxed. Are your ribs heavier to the floor than they were before? Is your low back curve closer to your pelvis?*

▶ *Finally, take a full breath and notice what areas of your torso expand when your lungs fill with air. Do you sense greater movement? Is it easier to take a deep breath?*

▶ *If you sense any of these changes, your body has returned to a more ideal position.*

Upper Body Length Sequence

Rest Assess

Gentle Rocking

Shoulder Blade Reach

Double Arm Reach

Rest Reassess

Rest Assess

▶ *Lie on the floor with your arms and legs straight and relaxed, palms face up. Take a breath and allow your body to relax into the floor.*

▶ *Remember, if all your upper back weight is on your shoulder blades, if your mid-back is arched off the floor, if your tailbone is more weighted than your butt cheeks, or if the backs of your thighs feel off the floor on one or both sides, you have identified stuck stress in your body.*

▶ *Close your eyes and, using your Body Sense, notice what you feel.*

▶ *Notice where your head is touching the floor. Is it tilted back? Does it feel off-center?*

▶ *Sense the lift of your neck. Does it feel curved or straight?*

▶ *Turn your head left and right. Do you feel pain or limited range? Do you sense any tightness in your neck?*

▶ *Notice your upper body. Ideally, your upper back is relaxed and resting on your ribs, or mid-back, and not your shoulder blades. Is one shoulder blade more weighted to the floor than the other? Do you feel the edge of either shoulder blade? Are your bottom ribs on or off the floor? Are your arms balanced from left to right?*

▶ *Finally, take a full breath and notice what areas of your torso expand when your lungs fill with air. Does your belly move? Ribs? Both? Just sense what moves and what doesn't.*

▶ *Take note of what you feel so you can compare after you complete the Upper Body Length Sequence.*

Gentle Rocking

▶ *Sit next to the bottom of the roller and lean away from it. Put your hands behind you, then shift your weight so that you're on top of the roller. Make sure your knees are bent and your feet are flat on the floor, approximately hip-width apart.*

▶ *Using your hands for support, slowly roll yourself down along the length of the roller.*

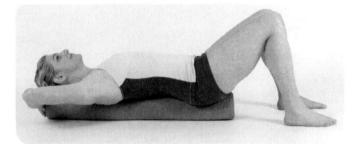

▶ *Touch the top of your head to make sure it is fully supported by the roller. Make sure your pelvis is on the roller.*

▶ *Place your forearms on the floor and take a breath.*

▶ *Allow your head, chest, and pelvis to slowly tip toward the floor on one side. Then come back through the center and slowly tip toward the other side. You want to get a sense of gently falling and catching* 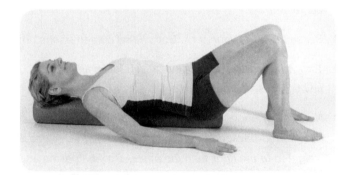 *yourself with your forearm, while keeping the back of your head, your spine, and the center of your pelvis aligned and heavy on the roller at all times. Continue to gently rock from left to right for about 30 seconds.*

▶ *Notice what you feel. Do you tip your body more easily to one side than to the other?*

Shoulder Blade Reach

▶ *Place your hands on the sides of your ribs with your elbows on the floor.*

▶ *Straighten out your arms and extend them toward the ceiling, palms facing in, with your shoulder blades weighted and heavy around the roller. Your hands should remain over your lower ribs, not directly above your shoulders.*

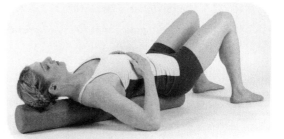

▶ *Breathe in, keep your arms straight and energized, and without shrugging your shoulders, reach your fingertips toward the ceiling.*

▶ *On the exhale, allow the weight of your arms to slowly sink your shoulder blades down around the roller without bending your elbows.*

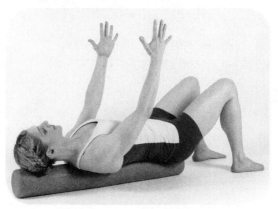

▶ *Breathe in and reach your arms up again without shrugging.*

Notice if you tend to shrug your shoulders or move your ribs as you create the movement, or if one of your shoulder blades touches the roller more than the other one when you release them around the roller.

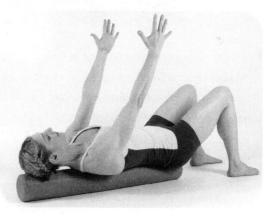

If you sense any clicking or discomfort while creating this movement, slow down or make the movement smaller.

▶ *Repeat this 5–10 times.*

Double Arm Reach

▶ *Place your hands on the sides of your ribs, elbows on the floor. Open your forearms away from your torso to make a letter W.*

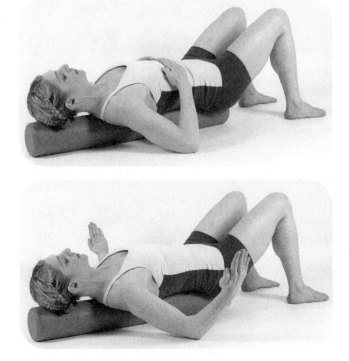

▶ *Lift your elbows off the floor as you reach your fingertips away from the center of your chest without shrugging your shoulders, locking your elbows, or lifting your ribs off the roller. Your hands are just above your body. Your arms are in line with your ribs, rather than straight out from your shoulders.*

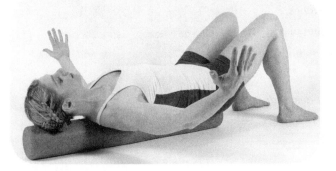

- *Keeping your palms face up, slowly extend one wrist and point your fingertips toward the floor as you flex the other wrist and point your fingertips toward the ceiling.*

  Keep your pelvis and ribs heavy on the roller, and keep your core engaged.

- *Switch sides. Slowly extend the other wrist as you point your other fingertips toward the ceiling.*

- *Take focused breaths into your chest as you flex and extend your wrists in opposition 6–10 times. Notice the pull across the front of your upper body, from fingertip to fingertip.*

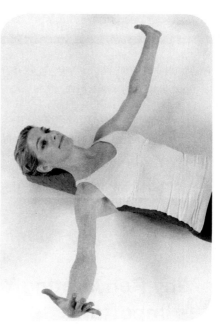

  I call this flossing the nerves. This technique creates a gentle tensional pull that rehydrates the tissues around the nerves and blood vessels, which are frequently compressed, decreasing blood flow, the strength of your grip, and finger dexterity and causing wrist and arm pain.

- *Try this same motion while making fists. This is great for hydrating the tissues of the wrist itself. You can also open your hands again and try turning your palms face down to flex and extend the wrists with open palms and then closed fists. Notice how the tensional pull in your arms changes.*

Rest Reassess

- *Lie on the floor with your arms and legs straight and relaxed, palms face up. Breathe and allow your body to relax into the floor. Close your eyes and take a moment to reassess.*

- *Remember the four common imbalances. Did you make changes? Do your ribs feel more weighted to the floor? Is your low back curve more relaxed and closer to your pelvis? Is your pelvis more weighted on your butt cheeks than on your tailbone? Have the backs of your thighs settled to the floor?*

- *Turn your head from left to right. Do you have more range of motion? Is there less pain or stiffness as you turn your head?*

- *Notice whether your upper body is more relaxed. Are your ribs heavier to the floor than they were before? Is your low back curve closer to your pelvis?*

- *Finally, take a full breath and notice what areas of your torso expand when your lungs fill with air. Do you sense greater movement? Is it easier to take a deep breath?*

- *If you sense any of these changes, you have alleviated stuck stress in your body.*

▶ Why Rehydrating Your Upper Body Is Important

Ease of movement in your upper body, specifically your ribs and shoulders, is important whether you need to turn your head to look out your car window, reach your arm up to a high shelf, bend over to pick up something, or take a walk. Without ease of movement of your shoulder blades and the space in between each and every rib, the areas above and below—your neck and low back—become compressed. In fact, stuck stress in the ribs is often the source of pain in these two spaces.

When you have pain in your neck or low back, you might stretch or massage the area to try to relieve the tension and discomfort. However, as long as stuck stress and fixation remain in your upper and mid-back, the compression in your neck and low back cannot be fully resolved, no matter what you do.

What causes the loss of movement in your upper back? In addition to repetitive movements and postures, circumstances such as asthma, heart conditions, pregnancy, large breasts, and chronic emotional states can cause stuck stress and fixation.

Restoring the fluid state around and within the ribs and shoulder girdle can help relieve stuck stress in the neck, upper back, and low back. Indeed, rehydrating this region dramatically improves the tensional energy of your entire body, which results in better alignment, movement, and function. In addition to pain relief, improvement in lung volume, organ function, upper back strength, and low back and neck mobility can be achieved through self-treatment with MELT.

▶ Your MELT Rehydrate Plan

Continue to do the Upper or Lower Body Compression and Length Sequences one to three times a week in the evening to restore tensional energy and to erase stuck stress. As you become proficient at Rehydrating, you will be able to do these sequences more quickly and easily. But be sure not to rush. Remember, to create a rehydration effect, connective tissue needs gentle compression and slow movements.

And, of course, make sure to drink water before and after you MELT. These MELT moves draw fresh fluid into the tissues that surround your muscles and joints—but this can't happen unless you drink enough water!

Continue to do your Rebalance Sequence and the Hand and/or Foot Treatment three times a week or more, either with the Upper or Lower Body Compression and Length Sequences or separately. You are on your way toward MELTing ten minutes, three times a week.

With MELT, you are in charge of your self-treatment. How will you know when to move on? Your self-assessments. When you reassess, do you sense any of the described body changes? You may notice immediate changes the first time you do the sequence, or it could take a few weeks. Once you notice these changes in your body, pay attention to how you feel the next day. Do you sense greater body ease or flexibility? Do you notice a reduction in stiffness, discomfort, or pain? These lasting changes indicate that your Autopilot is responding to your self-treatment and becoming more efficient.

Once you can sense lasting change from the Rehydration sequences, you are ready to move on to the next step, Releasing your neck and low back.

Oh, and did I mention to keep drinking water?

12

Release the Neck and Low Back

You are becoming a Hands-Off Bodyworker and creating powerful changes in your
body. Your joints are less stiff upon waking. You have less discomfort or pain. You
have greater body ease and flexibility. Your sleep is more restful and restorative. You
may have noticed an improvement in your overall energy and mood.

These changes mean that your body is responding to your self-treatment with
MELT. These changes will last and will likely increase as you continue to take care of
yourself in this new way. If you have yet to experience any of these changes, keep
MELTing and drinking water. The changes will come. Everyone's body is different.
Give your body time, and it will respond to your self-treatment.

At this point, your stuck stress is reduced, your Body Sense is heightened, and
your tensional energy is more cohesive. Perhaps most important, your Autopilot is
operating more efficiently—it can more easily find your center of gravity and your
joints. Your reflexive grounding and core stabilizing mechanisms are in better communication. Your body's natural healing capabilities are heightened.

You created these changes on your own by Reconnecting, Rebalancing, and
Rehydrating. This shows that your body is adaptable—a key element in achieving and
sustaining a more youthful, healthy body. It's exciting. You are improving your current
state of health and reducing the negative effects we associate with aging. And it's only
the beginning.

Now you are ready to address the final systemic effect of the accumulation of stuck
stress—the loss of joint space in your neck and/or low back. If you have neck or low

back pain and stiffness, you may be wondering why you haven't addressed these areas yet. The reality is, you have. The Hand and Foot Treatment and the Rebalance and Rehydrate sequences have been restoring the fluid state of the connective tissue in your neck and low back and improving the internal communication needed to effectively self-treat these areas. This is what your neck and low back have been missing.

Try the following Release sequences in the evening, up to an hour before bedtime. Try the Neck Release Sequence one evening and the Low Back Release Sequence another. Do these sequences one or two times per week. When possible, do the corresponding compression sequences from the last chapter before doing the Release sequence. For example, do the Upper Body Compression Sequence before the Neck Release Sequence. For even greater results, add the corresponding length sequence as well. Continue to do your Rebalance sequence and Hand and/or Foot Treatment one to three times a week.

Remember to drink water before and after you MELT, and don't lie on the roller or keep the roller under any body part for more than ten minutes.

You'll know you're ready to move on to the MELT maps—a series of sequences—in the next chapter when you can do the Hand and Foot Treatment and the Rebalance Sequence, Upper and Lower Body Compression and Length Sequences, and the Neck and Low Back Release Sequences without relying on the instructions. This might take you a few weeks or a few months. There's nothing to be gained by rushing, so take your time. The systems you are self-treating respond best to focused, gentle, slow movement. Track your progress and amaze yourself with the changes you can make in just minutes a day.

Neck Release Sequence

Neck Turn Assess	**Neck Decompress**
Base of Skull Shear	**Neck Turn Reassess**

Neck Turn Assess

▶ *Lie on your back with your legs extended. You can bend your knees if lying with your legs straight causes unnecessary tension in your back. Be comfortable as you assess.*

▶ *Use your Body Sense to notice the curve of your neck. Without touching your neck, notice the shape and size of your neck space. Ideally, the highest point of the neck curve is closer to your head than to your shoulders.*

▶ *Slowly turn your head to the right and then to the left, keeping your chin away from your shoulders. Do you feel like you're able to turn your head more in either direction? Do you feel any pain or tension? Does it feel like your shoulders move when you turn your head?*

▶ *Take note of what you feel so you can compare after you Release your neck.*

Base of Skull Shear

▶ *Lie on your right side and rest the base of your skull, just behind your ear, on the top of the roller. Bend your knees and reach your right arm out so your shoulders are relaxed.*

▶ *Take a focused breath and begin creating small head circles in either direction 5–6 times to Shear the base of your skull. Then pause for a moment, take a focused breath, and allow this area to sink further into the roller.*

▶ Open your left knee toward the ceiling so you're lying on the right half of your back. The roller is still under the base of your skull on the right side, an inch or so away from your ear, closer to the center of the base of your skull.

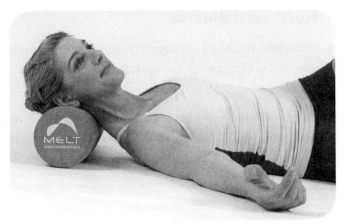

▶ Repeat the circles to Shear. Pause and take a focused breath.

▶ Turn onto your left side and repeat the Shear on the left side. In each spot, pause and take a focused breath.

▶ Lie on your back with your knees bent and rest the center of the base of your skull on the roller. Lift your chin slightly.

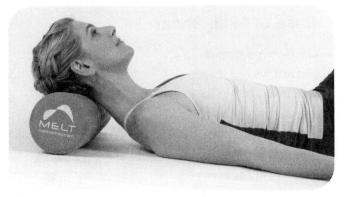

▶ While maintaining consistent pressure, create small figure 8 motions on the center of the base of your skull 5–6 times. Keep your pressure constant and your chin slightly lifted. Pause and take a focused breath.

Neck Decompress

▶ *Keep your knees bent, place your hands on the roller, and push the roller up about 1 inch toward the center of the back of your head. Take your hands away from the roller. Tip your nose toward the ceiling and apply gentle pressure on top of the roller. You must maintain consistent pressure throughout this move.*

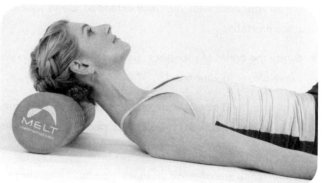

▶ *Inhale and, on the exhale, slowly nod your chin down slightly.*

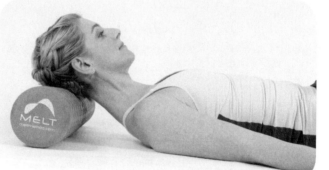

▶ *Inhale as you hold this position and, on the exhale, lift your chin slightly and return your nose toward the ceiling. Pause on the inhale; move on the exhale.*

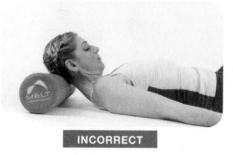

INCORRECT

You are not trying to touch your chin to your chest. The movement you create should be small and slow. Notice if your shoulders lift as you tip your head upward. Keep your upper back still and relaxed.

▶ *Repeat this head nod 4 times, pausing on the inhale, moving on the exhale.*

▶ *Remove the roller from the back of your head and gently bring your head to the floor.*

Neck Turn Reassess

▶ *Lie on your back with your legs extended. Bend your knees if your back is uncomfortable.*

▶ *Sense the curve of your neck. Does it feel lighter? Do you notice a more distinct curve closer to your head?*

▶ *Turn your head slowly from left to right. Do you have more range of motion? Is there less pain or stiffness in your neck? Are your back and shoulders more relaxed as you turn your head?*

▶ *If you sense any of these changes, you have decompressed your neck.*

Low Back Release Sequence

Rest Assess

Low Back Decompress

SI Joint Shear

Rest Reassess

Pelvic Tuck and Tilt Challenge

Rest Assess

▶ *Lie on the floor with your arms and legs straight and relaxed, palms face up. Take a breath and allow your body to relax into the floor.*

▶ *Remember, if all your upper back weight is on your shoulder blades, if your mid-back is arched off the floor, if your tailbone is more weighted than your butt cheeks, or if the backs of your thighs feel off the floor on one or both sides, you have identified stuck stress in your body.*

▶ *Close your eyes and, using your Body Sense, notice what you feel.*

▶ *Notice in particular the curve of your low back. Where do you feel the peak of the curve? Does it feel like it's above or below your belly button? Are your bottom ribs on or off the floor? Does it feel like there's a big curve up toward your shoulder blades or perhaps there is no curve at all?*

Take note of what you feel so you can compare after you Release your low back.

SI Joint Shear

▶ *Engage your core, lift your hips, and place your pelvis on top of the roller.*

▶ *Bring both knees toward your chest. The roller should not slip out, nor should you feel like the roller is under your low back.*

If you have a hard time getting your pelvis in the correct position, place a folded towel or yoga mat underneath your head and upper back.

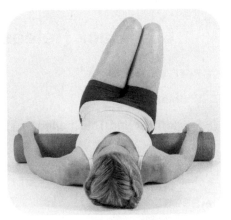

▶ *Keep your knees fully bent and your inner thighs together, and relax your lower legs and feet. Keep your core engaged and your ribs relaxed and heavy on the floor.*

▶ *Slowly move your knees away from your chest so your knees aim toward the ceiling, but stop before your thighs are fully perpendicular to the roller. This will help keep your low back relaxed.*

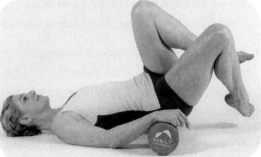

▶ *Maintain a consistent pressure and slowly tip your legs slightly right and left between the one and eleven o'clock positions to explore both SI joints.*

Remember, don't angle your knees too far to either side. Your goal is for your weight to be on the back of the pelvis, not on your hips.

As you move, try not to arch your back or move your ribs. Focus on moving your pelvis and not your ribs by keeping your core engaged.

▶ *Pause on the right side and Shear the right SI joint by making small circles with both knees 2–3 times in each direction.*

▶ *Then try circling just the leg you're leaning toward in slightly larger but slower circles. Also try slowly moving your knees forward and back in a marching motion 2–3 times.*

▶ *Keep your legs tipped to the right side, pause for a moment, maintain the pressure, and take 2 focused breaths.*

▶ *Return your knees to the center and repeat on the left side.*

Pelvic Tuck and Tilt Challenge

▶ *With your pelvis on the roller, place your palms on the front of your thighs, close to your knees. Gently push your knees away from your chest until your arms are straight. Keep your thighs angled slightly toward your side of the roller. Make sure your legs are relaxed and knees fully bent.*

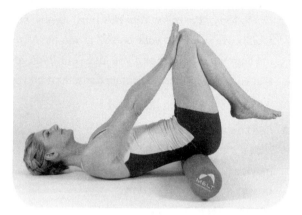

▶ *Take a focused breath and actively sink your ribs toward the floor below your shoulder blades. Keep your shoulders relaxed.*

▶ *Breathe in and, on the exhale, gently press your thighs into your hands as if you were trying to bring your knees to your chest, but don't bend your elbows or shrug your shoulders. Feel the subtle engagement deep within your abdomen. If you feel fatigue in the front of your thighs, you are pressing too hard.*

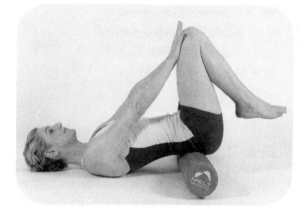

▶ *Keep your mid ribs weighted to the floor by keeping your core engaged.*

▶ *Take a breath in and, on the exhale, try to tuck your pelvis toward your side of the roller, keeping the pressure from your thighs to your hands constant and your arms straight. This movement will bring your pubic bone toward the belly button. As you tuck, your knees should rise slightly toward the ceiling as your arms resist movement toward your chest.*

▶ *Inhale while sustaining the pressure of your thighs toward your hands, and then on the exhale, slowly tilt your pelvis so the back of your pelvis is now weighted on the top of the roller. Your ribs must remain stable, but your low back will lift slightly, very close to your pelvis, as you tilt. Notice if your ribs have lifted from the floor when you tilt or if you lose your thigh-to-hand pressure. It is important that your thigh pressure remain consistent on your hands through both the tuck and the tilt!*

▶ *Keeping the pressure constant, repeat the tuck and tilt 4–5 times, moving slowly. The movement is be very subtle if you perform it correctly. Don't exaggerate the tilt.*

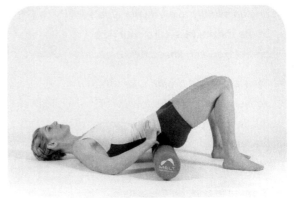

The first few times you try this move, practice tucking and tilting your pelvis with your feet on the floor. Remember to keep your ribs stable.

Low Back Decompress

▶ *Maintain the tilted position of your pelvis, with the back of your pelvis heavy on the top of the roller. Breathe in and, on the exhale, gently increase your thigh-to-hand pressure and sink the back of your ribs toward the floor without losing the tilt of your pelvis.*

▶ *Notice how much abdominal engagement is created by maintaining all three points of pressure—thighs to hands, mid-back toward the floor, and the back of the pelvis on top of the roller.*

▶ *Find your core with your sound (shhh, seee, or haaa) and sense the abdomen drawing inward as you sustain all three points of pressure.*

- *Inhale and subtly relax all three points of pressure, but don't change your position. When you exhale, re-engage the three points of pressure—thighs to hands, mid ribs to floor, pelvis to roller—without the sound. There is no visible movement throughout this part of the technique. Repeat one more time.*

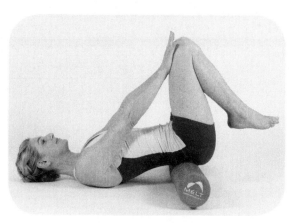

If you feel fatigue in the front of your thighs or hips, you are working too hard. Bring your thighs slightly closer to your head and try the sequence again.

- *Come off the roller and lie down on the floor on your back with your legs extended.*

Rest Reassess

- *Lie on the floor with your arms and legs straight and relaxed, palms face up. Breathe and allow your body to relax into the floor. Close your eyes and take a moment to reassess.*

- *Remember the four common imbalances. Did you make changes? Do your ribs feel more weighted to the floor? Is your low back curve more relaxed? Is your pelvis more weighted on your butt cheeks than on your tailbone? Have the backs of your thighs settled to the floor?*

- *Notice in particular the curve of your low back. Does it feel like the peak of the curve is lower? Are your bottom ribs closer to the floor? Does it feel like you have a distinct low back curve, closer to your pelvis?*

- *If you sense any of these changes, you have successfully decompressed your low back.*

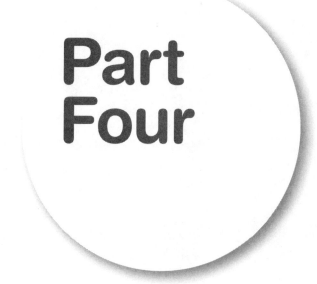

Part
Four

13

MELT Maps

Congratulations! You are now a Hands-Off Bodyworker. You have learned the language of MELT and mastered the Four R's. You have taken control of your health and longevity in ways you may not have thought possible. Other healthy habits, such as good nutrition, regular exercise, consistent water intake, and adequate sleep now yield a greater benefit.

Here are some other changes you may have noticed since you started MELTing:

- Your body is more comfortable during your day-to-day activities.

- Movement is more effortless, and you feel more stable and flexible.

- You feel more grounded and clearheaded.

- You can breathe with greater ease.

- You fall asleep more easily and sleep more soundly.

- You wake up more rested and have more vibrant energy throughout your day.

- You have fewer aches and pains, and a greater sense of overall well-being.

- You digest nutrients and eliminate waste easily.

- Your skin looks brighter and more supple.

- Your athletic endurance, performance, and recovery time have improved.

These are some of the most noticeable benefits of addressing your accumulated stuck stress and body-wide cellular dehydration. As you continue to MELT, you will experience more of these benefits and find that the improvements last longer. Your body will surprise you with its ability to renew itself.

These are very powerful, positive changes you are making. On a deeper level, a lot is going on to make this happen. By rehydrating your connective tissue and releasing stuck stress:

- You have transformed dehydrated tissue into healthy, hydrated tissue.

- You have restored the fluid state of the collagen matrix, which improves the tissue's extensibility, or elastic supportiveness.

- Your connective tissue system is better able to efficiently manage daily tension and compression.

- Your muscles can relax, as they're no longer responsible for "holding" your posture.

- The environment of every system and cell in your body is better supported.

- Your reflexive stability systems are more responsive and in better balance.

- You've reduced accumulated stress on your nervous system.

- Your internal communication travels more quickly and clearly.

- You've decreased damaging inflammation.

- Your joints are more buoyant, resilient, and stable, and your whole body is in better alignment.

▶ Welcome to the EZ Zone!

When you rehydrate your connective tissue and rebalance the stress and restore regulators, your Autopilot begins to operate more efficiently. This means your whole body starts to function at a more optimal level. You can do more while expending less energy. With energy to spare, your body can do more of the things you love again.

This more ideal state is what I call the Efficiency Zone, or the EZ Zone. The EZ Zone is the optimal range in which the Autopilot can effectively regulate and stabilize all the other systems of the body, using minimal energy. When your Autopilot is operating in the EZ Zone, the countless micro-adjustments it makes throughout your day return your body to balance—no matter how stressful or demanding your day was.

The EZ Zone is the environment necessary for daily repair and healing, which means your body has less stuck stress and pain to manage. The repetitive stress and strain of day-to-day living no longer accumulates, even on the days when you don't MELT. This is how your body functioned when you were younger. MELT turns back the clock for your body.

By addressing the four effects of stuck stress, you have helped your Autopilot return to the EZ Zone. When you MELT, you also give your restore regulator the opportunity to be dominant while you are awake. This boosts your body's ability to heal itself and eliminate chronic pain and other symptoms.

MELT is also your tool to *stay* in the EZ Zone! In just ten minutes three times a week, you can support your body's ongoing maintenance and catch underlying issues before pain and other symptoms arise. By getting back in the EZ Zone and staying there, you have opened the door to optimal health, energy, vitality, and longevity—without pain.

▶ Your Self-Treatment Plan

Now you are ready to take what you've learned and start to mix and match sequences. Now that you are familiar with the moves, the instructions for the sequences on the following pages have been shortened for quick reference. The pictures will remind you where your body should be in relationship to the roller or ball. For the full instructions, you can always refer to Chapters 10–12.

Mixing and matching sequences creates a MELT map. A map combines a series of sequences to create a complete self-treatment that includes all Four R's: Reconnect, Rebalance, Rehydrate, and Release. This means that every time you MELT, you're addressing all four effects of stuck stress.

This chapter contains nine ten-minute maps and seven fifteen- to twenty-minute maps. In the beginning, it may take you longer than that amount of time to complete these maps. As you become more familiar with the sequences, you'll be able to do these maps more quickly and easily. Be sure not to rush.

Remember, ten minutes is the maximum amount of time you should compress any one area of your body on the roller. You can always come off the roller, reassess, and go back to what you were doing.

To maintain the changes you've created, MELT three times a week for ten minutes. That's the minimum. This method is so gentle, you can MELT every day if you like.

To get the best results and continue to make changes in your body, it's important to incorporate variety into your weekly MELT routine. To do this, pick two or three different maps to do every week, and don't repeat the same map twice in a row.

Try all of these maps. You will find that some maps yield a greater result for you than others—you'll notice the difference both when you reassess and the next day. It's great to identify what your favorite maps are and to do them more frequently. Go ahead and pick a few and rotate them to get the best results and avoid falling into a self-treatment rut.

Until this point, I have asked you to MELT in the evening, if possible, to support your Autopilot. Now I want you to feel free to MELT at different times of the day to find out what works best for you. Try MELTing upon rising, after work, before and/or after exercise, as long as it's at least an hour before bedtime. See what works best for your body and your schedule.

Continue to drink a glass of water before and after every MELT map. And just in case, keep a glass of water close by during your treatment.

To find videos (including the Hand and Foot Treatment DVD and the MELT Method DVD) or an instructor or class near you, go to www.meltmethod.com.

▶ Maps

The MELT maps are outlined on the next two pages. Following the maps you will find a chart that will help you locate the instructions for the sequences within each map.

Ten-Minute Maps

❶ **Soft Ball Hand or Foot Treatment**
Rebalance and Upper Body Length Sequence

---

❷ **Soft Ball Hand and Foot Treatment**

---

❸ **Mini Soft Ball Hand Treatment**
Mini Soft Ball Foot Treatment
Rebalance and Upper Body Length Sequence

---

❹ **Mini Soft Ball Hand Treatment**
Rebalance and Upper Body Length Sequence
Neck Release Sequence

---

❺ **Mini Soft Ball Hand Treatment**
Upper Body Compression Sequence
Rebalance and Upper Body Length Sequence

---

❻ **Mini Soft Ball Foot Treatment**
Lower Body Length and Low Back Release Sequence

---

❼ **Mini Soft Ball Foot Treatment**
Lower Body Compression Sequence
Neck Release Sequence

---

❽ **Rebalance and Upper Body Length Sequence**
Neck Release Sequence

---

❾ **Rebalance and Upper Body Length Sequence**
Lower Body Length and Low Back Release Sequence

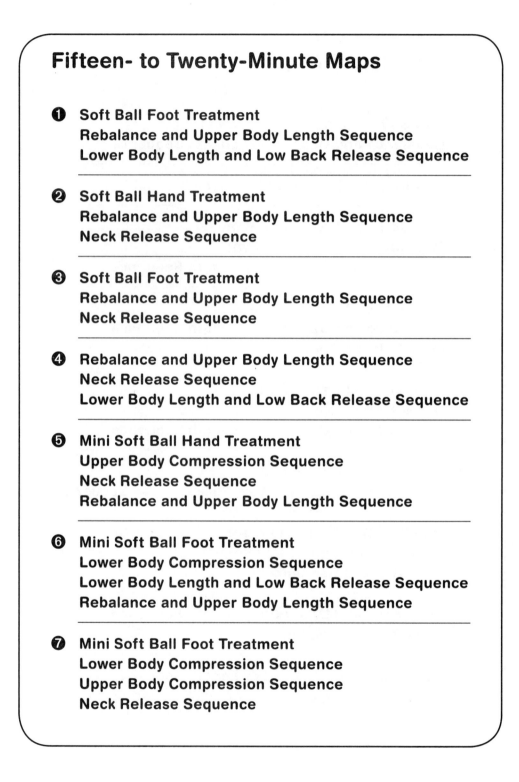

Fifteen- to Twenty-Minute Maps

❶ **Soft Ball Foot Treatment**
Rebalance and Upper Body Length Sequence
Lower Body Length and Low Back Release Sequence

---

❷ **Soft Ball Hand Treatment**
Rebalance and Upper Body Length Sequence
Neck Release Sequence

---

❸ **Soft Ball Foot Treatment**
Rebalance and Upper Body Length Sequence
Neck Release Sequence

---

❹ **Rebalance and Upper Body Length Sequence**
Neck Release Sequence
Lower Body Length and Low Back Release Sequence

---

❺ **Mini Soft Ball Hand Treatment**
Upper Body Compression Sequence
Neck Release Sequence
Rebalance and Upper Body Length Sequence

---

❻ **Mini Soft Ball Foot Treatment**
Lower Body Compression Sequence
Lower Body Length and Low Back Release Sequence
Rebalance and Upper Body Length Sequence

---

❼ **Mini Soft Ball Foot Treatment**
Lower Body Compression Sequence
Upper Body Compression Sequence
Neck Release Sequence

◗ Sequence Guide

Use the At-a-Glance Instructions for the sequences referenced in the Maps on the previous two pages. These instructions contain shortened descriptions and a single photograph for each move. If you want to see the full instructions for a move, refer to the page numbers in the right-hand column. To see the moves in action, refer to the MELT Method DVD, available at www.meltmethod.com.

At-a-Glance Instructions	Long Instructions
Rebalance and Upper Body Length Sequence (p. 232)	Rebalance Sequence (p. 82) Upper Body Length Sequence (p. 203)
Upper Body Compression Sequence (p. 236)	Upper Body Compression Sequence (p. 194)
Lower Body Compression Sequence (p. 241)	Lower Body Compression Sequence (p. 174)
Neck Release Sequence (p. 246)	Neck Release Sequence (p. 123)
Lower Body Length and Low Back Release Sequence (p. 248)	Lower Body Length Sequence (p. 186) Low Back Release Sequence (p. 217)
Soft Ball Foot Treatment (p. 253)	Soft Ball Foot Treatment (p. 162)
Soft Ball Hand Treatment (p. 256)	Soft Ball Hand Treatment (p. 167)
Mini Soft Ball Foot Treatment (p. 260)	Mini Soft Ball Foot Treatment (p. 140)
Mini Soft Ball Hand Treatment (p. 262)	Mini Soft Ball Hand Treatment (p. 137)

Rebalance and Upper Body Length Sequence

Rest Assess	3-D Breath
Gentle Rocking	Shoulder Blade Reach
Pelvic Tuck and Tilt	Double Arm Reach
3-D Breath Breakdown	Rest Reassess

Rest Assess

▶ *Lie on the floor with your arms and legs straight and relaxed, palms face up. Take a breath and allow your body to relax into the floor.*

▶ *Remember, if all your upper back weight is on your shoulder blades, if your mid-back is arched off the floor, if your tailbone is more weighted than your butt cheeks, or if the backs of your thighs feel off the floor on one or both sides, you have identified stuck stress in your body.*

▶ *Close your eyes and, using your Body Sense, notice what you feel.*

▶ *Turn your head left and right. Do you feel pain or limited range?*

▶ *Assess your Autopilot. Imagine splitting yourself into right and left sides. Notice if one side of your body feels more on the floor than the other. Does the right or the left side feel heavier or longer, or do they feel even?*

▶ *Finally, breathe and notice if there are any restrictions as you take a full breath.*

Gentle Rocking

▶ *Lie along the length of the roller.*

▶ *Place your forearms on the floor and take a focused breath.*

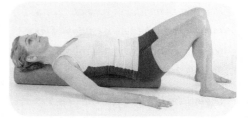

▶ *Allow your head, chest, and pelvis to slowly tip toward the floor on one side. Then come back through the center and slowly tip toward the other side. You want to get a sense of gently falling and catching yourself with your forearm, while keeping the back of your head, your spine, and the center of your pelvis aligned and heavy on the roller at all times. Continue to gently rock from left to right for about 30 seconds.*

Pelvic Tuck and Tilt

▶ *Come back to the center. Make sure your feet are still in line with your sits bones.*

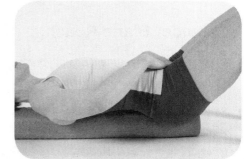

▶ *Place your hands on the front of your pelvis, fingertips on your pubic bone and the heels of your hands on your front hip bones.*

▶ *Slowly tuck and tilt your pelvis 5–6 times, keeping your ribs stable and your foot pressure constant.*

3-D Breath Breakdown

▶ *Take 4–5 focused breaths in each direction—front to back, side to side, and top to bottom—allowing the diaphragm to expand in two directions as you inhale.*

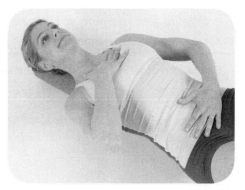

3-D Breath

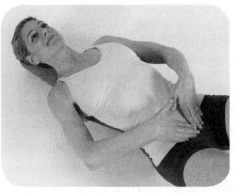

▶ *Place both hands on your belly and take a breath into all six sides of your torso, expanding three-dimensionally. Try this 2–3 times.*

▶ *During the next exhale, make a firm* shhh, seee, *or* haaa *sound and sense the reflexive action in your deep abdomen. Repeat 3–4 times.*

▶ *Then, without using the sound, see if you can use your Body Sense to feel and follow that same reflexive action. Try this 2–3 times.*

Shoulder Blade Reach

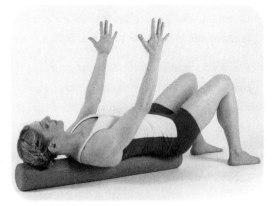

▶ *Place your hands on the sides of your ribs with your elbows on the floor.*

▶ *Straighten out your arms and extend them toward the ceiling, palms facing in, with your shoulder blades weighted and heavy around the roller. Your hands should remain over your lower ribs, not directly above your shoulders.*

▶ *Breathe in, keep your arms straight and energized, and without shrugging your shoulders, reach your fingertips toward the ceiling.*

▶ *On the exhale, allow the weight of your arms to slowly sink your shoulder blades down around the roller without bending your elbows.*

▶ *Breathe in and reach your arms up again without shrugging.*

▶ *Repeat this 5–10 times.*

Double Arm Reach

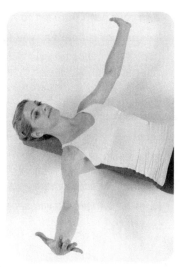

▶ *Place your hands on the sides of your ribs, elbows on the floor. Open your forearms away from your torso to make a letter W.*

▶ *Lift your elbows off the floor as you reach your fingertips away from the center of your chest without shrugging your shoulders, locking your elbows, or lifting your ribs off the roller. Your hands are just above your body. Your arms are in line with your ribs, rather than straight out from your shoulders.*

▶ *Keeping your palms face up, slowly extend one wrist and point your fingertips toward the floor as you flex the other wrist and point your fingertips toward the ceiling.*

▶ *Switch sides. Take focused breaths into your chest as you slowly flex and extend your wrists in opposition 6–10 times. Notice the pull across the front of your upper body, from fingertip to fingertip.*

▶ *Try this same motion while making fists. You can also open your hands again and try turning your palms face down to flex and extend the wrists with open palms and then closed fists.*

▶ *Put your hands on the floor and slowly come off the roller by straightening out one leg and sliding off that side, first with your pelvis, and then your ribs and head.*

Rest Reassess

▶ *Lie on the floor with your arms and legs straight and relaxed, palms face up. Breathe and allow your body to relax into the floor. Close your eyes and take a moment to reassess.*

▶ *Remember the four common imbalances. Did you make changes? Do your ribs feel more weighted to the floor? Is your low back curve more relaxed and closer to your pelvis? Is your pelvis more weighted on your butt cheeks than on your tailbone? Have the backs of your thighs settled to the floor?*

▶ *Turn your head from left to right. Do you have more range of motion? Is there less pain or stiffness as you turn your head?*

▶ *Notice whether your upper body is more relaxed. Are your ribs heavier to the floor than they were before? Is your low back curve closer to your pelvis?*

▶ *Assess your Autopilot. When you divide yourself into right and left sides, do the sides feel more even? Does it feel like there's less of a distinction between your left and right halves?*

▶ *Finally, take a full breath and notice what areas of your torso expand when your lungs fill with air. Do you sense greater movement? Is it easier to take a deep breath?*

Upper Body Compression Sequence

Rest Assess   **Upper Back Rinse**

Rib Length Assess   **Rib Length Reassess**

Upper Back Glide and Shear   **Rest Reassess**

Shoulder Blade Glide and Shear

Rest Assess

▶ *Lie on the floor with your arms and legs straight and relaxed, palms facing up. Take a breath and allow your body to relax into the floor.*

▶ *Remember, if all your upper back weight is on your shoulder blades, if your mid-back is arched off the floor, if your tailbone is more weighted than your butt cheeks, or if the backs of your thighs feel off the floor on one or both sides, you have identified stuck stress in your body.*

▶ *Close your eyes and, using your Body Sense, notice what you feel.*

▶ *Turn your head left and right. Do you feel pain or limited range?*

- *Notice your upper body. Ideally, your upper back is relaxed and resting on your ribs, or mid-back, and not on your shoulder blades. Are your bottom ribs on or off the floor?*

- *Notice the curve of your low back. Does it feel like there's a big curve up toward your shoulder blades or perhaps there is no curve at all?*

Rib Length Assess

- *Rest your shoulder blades on the roller and bend your knees. Check that the bottom of your shoulder blades are on the foot side of the roller.*

- *Interlace your hands behind your head and let your neck relax. Tuck your pelvis. As you create the following movement, your core, low back, and neck remain still and stable.*

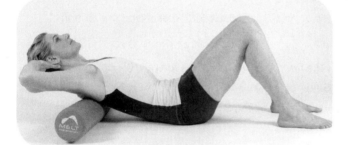

- *Breathe in. On the exhale, find your core, allow only your ribs to extend over the roller, and open your breastbone toward the ceiling.*

- *Take 2 focused breaths into your ribs and notice if you feel any stiffness in the front of your chest.*

- *Breathe in, and then on the exhale, curl your ribs forward to the starting position.*

- *Repeat the movement again. Are you able to move your ribs without moving your low back or neck?*

- *Repeat the movement again. This time, from the extended position, breathe in, and on your exhale, slowly side bend your ribs to the right. Take a focused breath into the left side of your ribs and notice the feeling as you breathe.*

On your next exhale, return your torso to the center and then slowly side bend to the left and take a focused breath. Does one side feel easier to breathe into?

▶ *Repeat one more time on each side. Notice if one or both sides feel restricted or if you move more to one side. Then return to the center.*

Upper Back Glide and Shear

▶ *Keep your hands behind your head for support and point your elbows toward the ceiling. Engage your core and lift your hips slightly off the floor to bring the roller to the top of your upper back. Keep your pelvis tucked.*

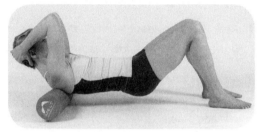

▶ *Push into your feet to gently Glide the roller up and down 2–3 inches of your upper back 6-8 times. Keep the motion small.*

▶ *Set your hips back down on the floor and curl your ribs forward slightly more. Take a focused breath and Shear by slowly side bending your upper body left and right in small movements 3 times, as if you are scratching an itch on your back. Keep your pressure constant.*

▶ *Return to the center, pause, and take a focused breath, letting your spine sink further into the roller.*

▶ *Lift your hips slightly off the ground, push into your feet to move the roller down your back 1–2 inches, and repeat the Glide and Shear. Pause and take a focused breath.*

▶ *Lift your hips and move the roller down 1–2 inches more, and then Glide and Shear. Pause and take a focused breath.*

Shoulder Blade Glide and Shear

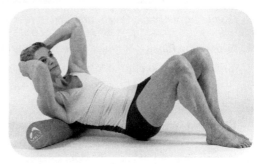

▶ *Rest your upper back on the roller with your hands behind your head, knees bent, feet flat on the floor. Keep your core engaged and tip your upper body slightly to the right so the roller is on the bottom of your right shoulder blade, not on your spine. Keep your back curled forward and lift your hips an inch off the floor.*

▶ *Using your feet, Glide up and down the bottom and inner edge of your right shoulder blade. If you find a tender spot, make your movement smaller and smaller and edge up against the area of stuck stress but don't land right on it.*

▶ *Set your right buttock on the floor. To Shear, release your right arm from behind your head and slowly create small circles or figure 8 movements with your arm in front of your body.*

▶ *Bring your hand back behind your head, pause, and take a focused breath.*

▶ *Return your body to the center. Then repeat these steps on the other shoulder blade.*

Upper Back Rinse

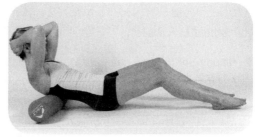

▶ *Find your core, set your feet slightly in front of your knees, and lift your hips an inch off the floor.*

▶ *Bring your knees over your feet so the roller moves to the upper part of your back. Take a focused breath.*

▶ *On the exhale, engage your core and gently push into your feet to allow the roller to slowly travel down your back with consistent, light pressure. Curl your ribs forward as your legs extend and your hips settle back to the floor.*

- ▶ *Reset your feet slightly in front of your knees and then find your core, lift your hips off the floor, and bring your knees over your feet again so the roller moves to your upper back. Pause and take a focused breath.*

- ▶ *Repeat the Rinse 3–4 times, then reset the roller under your shoulder blades and bend your knees.*

Rib Length Reassess

- ▶ *With the middle of your shoulder blades resting on top of the roller and your pelvis tucked, breathe in and then, on the exhale, allow only your ribs to extend over the roller again. Repeat once.*

- ▶ *Notice if you move more freely or sense a greater range of motion in this extended position. Repeat once.*

- ▶ *Maintain this extension, slowly side bend your ribs to the right, and take 2–3 focused breaths. Repeat on the left side.*

- ▶ *Repeat 2 times on each side.*

- ▶ *Notice if you move more freely or sense a greater range of motion when you side bend than you did before.*

Rest Reassess

- ▶ *Lie on the floor with your arms and legs straight and relaxed, palms face up. Breathe and allow your body to relax into the floor. Close your eyes and take a moment to reassess.*

- ▶ *Remember the four common imbalances. Did you make changes? Do your ribs feel more weighted to the floor? Is your low back curve more relaxed and closer to your pelvis? Is your pelvis more weighted on your butt cheeks than on your tailbone? Have the backs of your thighs settled to the floor?*

- ▶ *Turn your head from left to right. Do you have more range of motion? Is there less pain or stiffness as you turn your head?*

▶ *Notice whether your upper body is more relaxed. Are your ribs heavier to the floor than they were before? Is your low back curve closer to your pelvis?*

▶ *Finally, take a full breath and notice what areas of your torso expand when your lungs fill with air. Do you sense greater movement? Is it easier to take a deep breath?*

Lower Body Compression Sequence

Rest Assess

Back Thigh Shear

Calf Glide and Shear

Inner Thigh Glide and Shear

Calf Rinse

Inner and Back Thigh Rinse

Rest Reassess

Rest Assess

▶ *Lie on the floor with your arms and legs straight and relaxed, palms face up. Take a breath and allow your body to relax into the floor.*

▶ *Remember, if all your upper back weight is on your shoulder blades, if your mid-back is arched off the floor, if your tailbone is more weighted than your butt cheeks, or if the backs of your thighs feel off the floor on one or both sides, you have identified stuck stress in your body.*

▶ *Close your eyes and, using your Body Sense, notice what you feel.*

▶ *Turn your head left and right. Do you feel pain or limited range?*

▶ *Notice the curve of your low back. Does your back feel lifted off the floor from the navel to the shoulder blades?*

▶ *Notice if you sense your tailbone on the floor instead of your butt cheeks or if one side of your pelvis feels more weighted than the other.*

▶ *Feel whether your thighs are touching the floor and whether they feel equal.*

Back Thigh Shear

▶ *Place the roller underneath the backs of your thighs, just below the crease of your buttocks. Relax your legs and keep them heavy on the roller.*

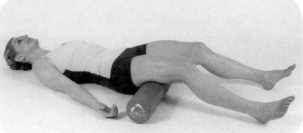

▶ *Slowly drag your legs together and apart to Shear the backs of the thighs 4–5 times.*

▶ *Bend one leg and relax it on the roller, and then drag and twist the other leg in and out 4–5 times. Repeat on the other thigh.*

▶ *Return your legs to the center, pause for 2 focused breaths, and allow your upper thighs to sink further into the roller.*

▶ *Move the roller halfway down your thighs and repeat the techniques, and then move it just above your knees and repeat.*

Calf Glide and Shear

▶ *Place the roller under the upper half of your right calf, and cross your left ankle over your right. Let your calf sink into the roller with tolerable pressure.*

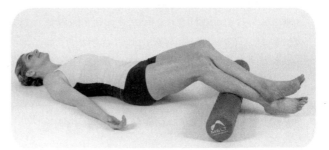

▶ *Slowly bend and straighten your knee 4–5 times to move the roller back and forth no more than 2 inches. Keep your feet and ankles relaxed, and maintain a consistent, tolerable pressure as you explore your calf for areas of stuck stress.*

▶ *Rotate your calf outward and repeat the small back-and-forth Gliding motion 3–4 times.*

- *Then rotate your calf inward and Glide 3–4 times.*

- *When you find an area of stuck stress, indirectly Shear by flexing and pointing your right ankle 3–4 times and then making circles with your ankle 3–4 times in each direction.*

- *Relax your ankle and create a direct Shear by turning your right leg in and out in a small, controlled movement, 1–2 inches, 4–5 times.*

- *Maintain compression and gently shift your leg slightly left to right, like you're scratching the calf against the roller.*

- *Pause, wait, and take 2 focused breaths while you let the calf sink into the roller.*

- *Move the roller down to the lower half of your right calf, a few inches above your ankle. Repeat the same Glide and Shear techniques in this region.*

- *Switch legs and repeat.*

Inner Thigh Glide and Shear

- *Lie on your right side and place the roller in front of you.*

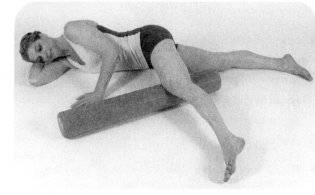

- *Place your left inner thigh on top of the roller, just above your knee. Push the top end of the roller away from you. Place your left hand on the floor.*

- *To Glide, allow your body to fall slightly forward. Then, using your left arm, push your body back so the roller moves 1–2 inches up and down your lower inner thigh, just above your knee, 4–5 times.*

- *To Shear, slowly bend and straighten the knee 3 times.*

- *Rotate the bent leg so your foot goes up and then down to the floor 3 times.*

▶ *Twist the flesh of your thigh against the roller in a slow scratching motion 3–4 times.*

▶ *Pause, wait, and take 2 focused breaths.*

▶ *Move the roller to the middle of your thigh and reset your body position. Rest your head on your right arm. Place your left hand on the floor.*

▶ *Repeat all of the techniques on this area.*

▶ *Move the roller up closer to your pelvis and repeat.*

▶ *Switch sides and repeat.*

Calf Rinse

▶ *Sit on the floor and place your arms behind you for support. With your right knee bent, rotate your right leg inward and place your inner ankle on the roller. Your foot is relaxed, and your big toe is close to the floor.*

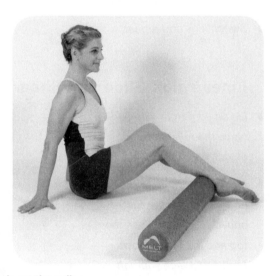

▶ *Lean forward and slowly straighten your right leg to allow the roller to move up your inner calf with consistent, light pressure. It's okay if the roller doesn't travel all the way up your calf.*

▶ *Rotate your leg so the back of your leg is on the roller.*

▶ *Lean back and slowly bend your knee to allow the roller to move down the back of your calf with consistent, light pressure. Stop before your ankle and repeat the Rinse 3–4 times.*

▶ *Repeat on the other leg.*

Inner and Back Thigh Rinse

▶ *Place your right inner thigh, just above the knee, on the left side of the roller.*

▶ *Use your arms to move your body forward, moving the roller toward the top of your inner thigh with consistent pressure.*

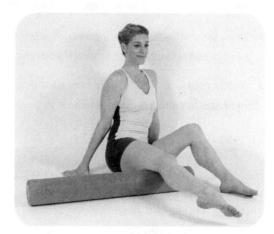

▶ *When you reach the top, think of twisting the flesh around the thigh bone as you rotate your leg so the back of your upper thigh is on the roller.*

▶ *Use your arms to move your body backward, moving the roller down your thigh with consistent pressure. Stop right above your knee.*

▶ *Again think of twisting the flesh around the thigh bone as you rotate your leg so that the inside of your thigh is on the roller. Slowly Rinse up the inner thigh with consistent pressure.*

▶ *Repeat this Rinsing pass 3–4 times.*

▶ *Repeat on the left thigh.*

Rest Reassess

▶ *Lie on the floor with your arms and legs straight and relaxed, palms face up. Breathe and allow your body to relax into the floor. Close your eyes and take a moment to reassess.*

▶ *Remember the four common imbalances. Did you make changes? Do your ribs feel more weighted to the floor? Is your low back curve more relaxed and closer to your pelvis? Is your pelvis more weighted on your butt cheeks than on your tailbone? Have the backs of your thighs settled to the floor?*

▶ *Turn your head from left to right. Do you have more range of motion? Is there less pain or stiffness as you turn your head?*

▶ *Bring your attention to your pelvis. If your tailbone was the most noticeable part of your pelvis on the floor, notice if you now sense your butt cheeks more.*

▶ *Notice your legs. Are the backs of your thighs more settled on the floor? Do the right and left sides feel more even?*

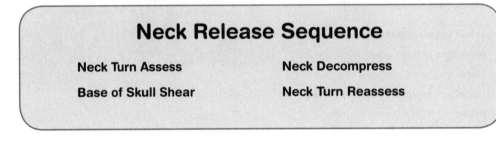

Neck Release Sequence

Neck Turn Assess   **Neck Decompress**

Base of Skull Shear   **Neck Turn Reassess**

Neck Turn Assess

▶ *Lie on the floor with your arms and legs straight and relaxed, palms face up. Bend your knees if your back is uncomfortable.*

▶ *Notice the curve of your neck. Ideally, the highest point of the neck curve is closer to your head than to your shoulders.*

▶ *Slowly turn your head to the right and then to the left, keeping your chin away from your shoulders. Do you feel like you're able to turn your head more in either direction? Do you feel any pain or tension? Does it feel like your shoulders move when you turn your head?*

Base of Skull Shear

▶ *Lie on your right side and rest the base of your skull, just behind your ear, on the top of the roller. Bend your knees and reach your right arm out so your shoulders are relaxed.*

- Take a focused breath and begin creating small head circles in either direction 5–6 times to Shear the base of your skull. Then pause for a moment, take a focused breath, and allow this area to sink further into the roller.

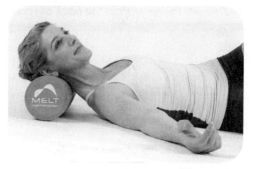

- Open your left knee toward the ceiling so you're lying on the right half of your back. The roller is still under the base of your skull on the right side, an inch or so away from your ear, closer to the center of the base of your skull.

- Repeat the circles to Shear. Pause and take a focused breath.

- Turn onto your left side and repeat the Shear on the left side. In each spot, pause and take a focused breath.

- Lie on your back with your knees bent and rest the center of the base of your skull on the roller. Lift your chin slightly.

- While maintaining consistent pressure, create small figure 8 motions on the center of the base of your skull 5–6 times. Keep your pressure constant and your chin slightly lifted. Pause and take a focused breath.

Neck Decompress

- Push the roller up about 1 inch toward the center of the back of your head. Tip your nose toward the ceiling and apply gentle pressure on top of the roller.

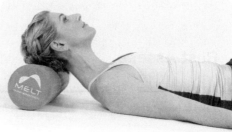

- Inhale and, on an exhale, slowly nod your chin slightly toward your chest.

- Inhale as you hold this position and, on the exhale, return your nose toward the ceiling. Pause on the inhale; move on the exhale.

- Repeat this head nod 4 times, pausing on the inhale, moving on the exhale.

▶ *Remove the roller from the back of your head and gently bring your head to the floor.*

Neck Turn Reassess

▶ *Lie on your back with your legs extended.*

▶ *Sense the curve of your neck. Does it feel lighter? Do you notice a more distinct curve closer to your head?*

▶ *Turn your head slowly from left to right. Do you have more range of motion? Is there less pain or stiffness in your neck? Are your back and shoulders more relaxed as you turn your head?*

Lower Body Length and Low Back Release Sequence

Rest Assess

SI Joint Shear

Bent Knee Press

Hip to Heel Press

Pelvic Tuck and Tilt Challenge

Low Back Decompress

Rest Reassess

Rest Assess

▶ *Lie on the floor with your arms and legs straight and relaxed, palms face up. Take a breath and allow your body to relax into the floor.*

▶ *Remember, if all your upper back weight is on the shoulder blades, if your mid-back is arched off the floor, if your tailbone is more weighted than your butt cheeks, or if the backs of your thighs feel off the floor on one or both sides, you have identified stuck stress that could be causing you unnecessary compression in your low back.*

- *Close your eyes and, using your Body Sense, notice what you feel.*

- *Take a second to notice the curve of your low back. Where do you feel the peak of the curve? Does it feel like it's above or below your belly button? Are your bottom ribs on or off the floor? Does it feel like there's a big curve up toward your shoulder blades or perhaps there is no curve at all?*

SI Joint Shear

- *Engage your core, lift your hips, and place your pelvis on top of the roller. Bring your knees into your chest to check the position of your pelvis on the roller.*

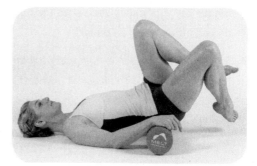

- *Point your knees toward the ceiling, but stop before your thighs are fully perpendicular to the roller.*

- *Slowly angle your knees slightly right and left to explore both SI joints. Try to keep your knees together.*

- *Pause on the right side and Shear the right SI joint by making small circles with your upper legs 2–3 times in each direction.*

- *Then try circling just the lower leg in larger but slower circles and slowly moving your knees forward and back in a marching motion, 2–3 times.*

- *Keep your legs tipped to the right side, pause for a moment, maintain the pressure, and take 2 focused breaths.*

- *Return your knees to the center and repeat on the left side.*

Bent Knee Press

- *With the roller still under your pelvis, place both feet on the floor, hip-width apart.*

- *Tuck your pelvis and allow your ribs to relax and sink into the floor.*

- *Engage your core. Lift your right leg up and interlace your hands over the shin or around the back of your thigh.*

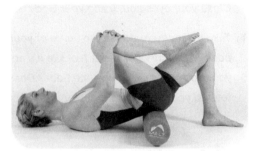

- *Keep your left foot firmly on the floor and keep your left knee in line with your hip. Make sure your hips remain level on top of the roller, from left to right.*

- *Inhale, and on the exhale, accentuate the tuck of your pelvis and sense the pull on the front of your left thigh. Take a focused breath as you pause.*

- *Inhale and relax, then exhale and tuck the pelvis as you draw your right knee toward your torso. Think about your left knee reaching over your left foot in the opposite direction. Take a focused breath. Repeat one more time on this side.*

- *Repeat on the other side.*

Hip to Heel Press

- *With the roller still under your pelvis, make sure your left foot is on the floor and your left knee is in line with your hip. Raise your right thigh so your knee points toward the ceiling.*

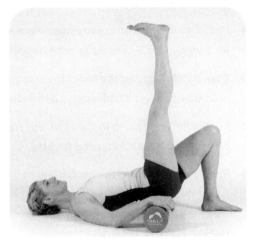

- *Straighten your right leg out in front of you and flex your ankle. Keep your pelvis heavy on top of the roller in a slight tilt, and keep your mid ribs relaxed and weighted to the floor.*

- *Keeping your leg straight, slowly bring your flexed right foot toward the ceiling and stop before your knee bends.*

- *On an exhale, in two directions, actively flex your ankle and tilt your pelvis, keeping your pelvis weighted to the top of the roller. Take a focused breath as you feel the tensional pull from your heel all the way down to your hip.*

- *Inhale and relax the foot. Then exhale and actively flex your foot and allow the pelvis to sink into the roller to find your tilt. Take a focused breath and pause as you accentuate the pull again. Repeat one more time on this side, then bring your right foot to the floor.*

- *Repeat on the other side.*

Pelvic Tuck and Tilt Challenge

- *Bring both knees toward your chest.*

- *Place your palms on the front of your thighs, close to your knees. Gently push your knees away from your chest until your arms are straight. Keep your thighs angled slightly toward your side of the roller.*

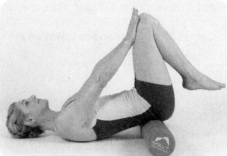

- *Take a focused breath and actively sink your ribs toward the floor below your shoulder blades.*

- *Breathe in and, on the exhale, gently press your thighs into your hands as if you were trying to bring your knees to your chest, but don't bend your elbows or shrug your shoulders.*

- *Take a breath in and, on the exhale, try to tuck your pelvis toward your side of the roller.*

- *Inhale while sustaining the pressure of your thighs toward your hands, and then on the exhale, slowly tilt your pelvis.*

- *Repeat the tuck and tilt 4–5 times, moving slowly.*

Low Back Decompress

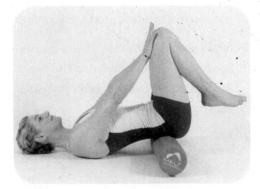

▶ *Maintain the tilted position of your pelvis. Breathe in and, on the exhale, gently increase your thigh-to-hand pressure and sink the back of your ribs toward the floor without losing the tilt of your pelvis.*

▶ *Inhale and subtly relax all three points of pressure, but don't change your position.*

▶ *On the exhale, re-engage the three points of pressure—thighs to hands, mid ribs to floor, pelvis to roller. Repeat one more time.*

▶ *Come off the roller and lie down on the floor on your back with your legs extended.*

Rest Reassess

▶ *Lie on the floor with your arms and legs straight and relaxed, palms face up. Breathe and allow your body to relax into the floor. Close your eyes and take a moment to reassess.*

▶ *Remember the four common imbalances. Did you make changes? Do your ribs feel more weighted to the floor? Is your low back curve more relaxed and closer to your pelvis? Is your pelvis more weighted on your butt cheeks than on your tailbone? Have the backs of your thighs settled to the floor?*

Soft Ball Foot Treatment

Body Scan Assess	Rinse
Autopilot Assess	Friction
Position Point Pressing	Body Scan Reassess
Glide	Final Body Scan Reassess
Shear	Autopilot Reassess

Body Scan Assess

▶ *Stand with your feet side by side, hip-width apart. Close your eyes and use your Body Sense to notice your feet. Use your Body Sense to scan up your legs. Notice the joints of your ankles, knees, and hips. Notice your muscles.*

Autopilot Assess

▶ *Keep your eyes closed and legs relaxed. Lift all ten toes off the floor and take three breaths. On the final exhale, set your toes down. Notice if you felt yourself drift forward. Try the same assessment with your eyes open and notice how much less you drift when you can rely on your sense of sight to remain balanced.*

Position Point Pressing

▶ *Stand up straight with your feet hip-width apart. Place the soft ball on the floor in front of you and step onto it so it aligns with position point 1.*

▶ *Put your feet side by side and gently shift some of your body weight onto the ball to create tolerable pressure.*

- *Then shift some of your weight off the ball. Repeat this shifting 2–3 times to ease into tolerable compression while you take focused breaths.*

- *Before you move to the next point, step backward with the opposite foot and shift your weight to that foot.*

- *Place the ball under position point 2, directly under the big toe knuckle.*

- *Gently rock forward to apply tolerable compression to that point.*

- *Step on your back foot to decompress the ball as you move to the next point.*

- *Continue this rocking motion as you compress and decompress each point.*

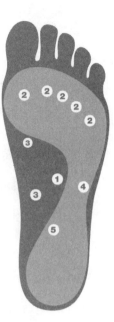

Glide

- *Place the ball on point 5, right in front of the heel. The ball of your foot and your toes are on the floor. Your heel is off the ground.*

- *Keeping the front of your foot on the floor, slowly move the ball from side to side in front of the heel.*

- *Continue Gliding the ball from side to side as you work your way to the back of the heel and then back to point 5.*

Shear

- *With the ball on point 5, use a slightly heavier compression to wiggle your foot left to right. The ball should barely move.*

Rinse

▶ *Place the ball on point 2, directly under the big toe knuckle.*

▶ *Keeping your heel on the floor, gently press the ball with consistent pressure across the knuckles, toward the outside of the foot. Lift your foot to return to the starting point and repeat 2 more times. Remember, you only Rinse in one direction.*

▶ *Place the ball on point 2 again, directly under the big toe knuckle. Press the ball toward your heel in a continuous motion with tolerable, consistent pressure.*

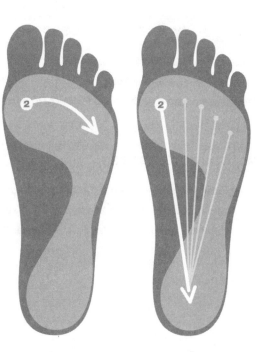

▶ *Lift your foot to move to the next knuckle. Repeat from each one.*

Friction

▶ *Using light, quick, random movements, rub your foot and toes over the ball in a scribble-like motion.*

Body Scan Reassess

▶ *When you finish this self-treatment on one foot, close your eyes and use your Body Sense to notice the side of the body you just self-treated.*

▶ *Notice your foot. Notice the joints of your leg. You may find that you don't sense the leg as separate parts and instead your leg feels more cohesive. Notice if you feel more grounded.*

Repeat all the techniques on the other foot.

Final Body Scan Reassess

▶ *Now that you've self-treated both sides of your body, close your eyes and use your Body Sense to feel your feet on the floor. Notice your joints. Do your legs feel more cohesive on both sides now? Do you feel more evenly grounded?*

Autopilot Reassess

▶ *With your eyes closed, repeat the Autopilot Assess, lifting your toes and setting them back down. Do you drift less when you set your toes back down than you did before you did the Soft Ball Foot Treatment?*

Soft Ball Hand Treatment

Wrist Assess	Rinse
Grip Assess	Finger Rinse
Finger Compression	Friction
Position Point Pressing	Wrist Reassess
Glide	Grip Reassess
Shear	

Wrist Assess

▶ *Bring your elbows and wrists together.*

▶ *Open your hands so that your palms face the ceiling. Ideally, your hands should look like the letter T. Notice if your hands look more like a Y or if your pinky finger bends.*

Grip Assess

▶ *Place a soft ball in one hand and squeeze it 3–4 times as firmly as you can.*

▶ *Then place the ball in the other hand and notice whether your grip feels equal in strength or if you have a stronger grip in one hand than in the other.*

Finger Compression

▶ *Press down on the ball with your index finger.*

▶ *Then decompress the ball and flex your index finger so your fingertip is touching the ball. Alternate between pressing the tip and the pad of your index finger 4 times. Repeat this motion with your other fingers and thumb.*

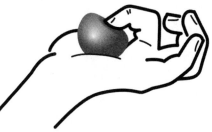

▶ *Switch hands and repeat.*

Position Point Pressing

▶ *Press your hand into the soft ball at each of the position points on the diagram, starting with point 1. Create a tolerable amount of pressure. You can use your other hand to create gentle compression.*

▶ *Then compress points 2–5. At each point, take a focused breath before lifting your hand and moving to the next point. Ease off pressure if you feel a strong sensation or pain. Take your time.*

▶ *Once you've pressed into each point, repeat on the other hand.*

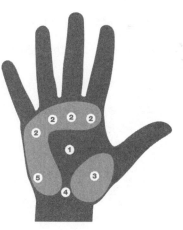

Glide

▶ *On your right hand, Glide the soft ball from point 3, across the base of the palm to point 5, and return to point 3 with consistent pressure. Keep the tip of your middle finger on the table or floor as you create the Glide.*

▶ *Continue back and forth as you take 3–4 focused breaths.*

▶ *Repeat on the left hand.*

Shear

▶ *Place the soft ball under point 3, the thumb pad, on your right hand and create small circles as you take 3–4 focused breaths. Move slowly and take your time with Shearing the thumb pad, as this area often carries a lot of stuck stress.*

▶ *Repeat on the left hand.*

Rinse

▶ *Starting at the tip of one finger on your right hand, slowly press the soft ball down the finger and across point 4 and over your wrist.*

▶ *Repeat, starting from each of the other fingers.*

▶ *Switch hands and repeat.*

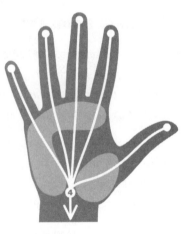

▶ *Next, start at the fingertip and slowly press the soft ball through your wrist and up your forearm in a continuous motion until you reach the elbow.*

▶ *Repeat, starting from each of the other fingers.*

▶ *Switch hands and repeat.*

Finger Rinse

▶ *Place your left hand flat on the floor or a table. Use the right hand to rub the soft ball over the top of and in between each finger of the left hand in one direction, from the knuckle to the nail. (This also stimulates point 4 on the top hand.)*

▶ *Repeat on the other hand.*

Friction

▶ *Using light, quick, random movements, rub one hand over the soft ball in a scribble-like motion. Be sure to include your fingers and wrists.*

▶ *Repeat on the other hand.*

Wrist Reassess

▶ *Bring your elbows and wrists together.*

▶ *Open your hands so that your palms face the ceiling. Do you feel a change in the flexibility of your wrists? Do you feel less tension in your arms? Do your fingers extend more fully?*

Grip Reassess

▶ *Remember what your grip strength felt like when you began and repeat the Grip Assess by squeezing the soft ball as firmly as you can 3–4 times in each hand. Can you create a more powerful grip with less effort? Does your grip feel more equal from left to right?*

Mini Soft Ball Foot Treatment

Body Scan Assess

Position Point Pressing

Glide

Shear

Rinse

Friction

Body Scan Reassess

Final Body Scan Reassess

Body Scan Assess

▶ *Stand with your feet side by side, hip-width apart. Close your eyes and use your Body Sense to notice your feet. Use your Body Sense to scan up your legs. Notice the joints of your ankles, knees, and hips. Notice if you have any tension in your legs.*

Position Point Pressing

▶ *Stand up straight with your feet hip-width apart. Place the soft ball on the floor in front of you and step onto it so it aligns with position point 1.*

▶ *Put your feet side by side and gently shift some of your body weight onto the ball to create tolerable pressure.*

▶ *Then shift some of your weight off the ball. Repeat this shifting 2–3 times to ease into tolerable compression while you take focused breaths.*

▶ *Step backward with the opposite foot and shift your weight to that foot.*

▶ *Place the ball under position point 5, in front of the heel bone. Apply tolerable compression to that point as you take a focused breath.*

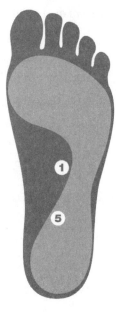

Glide

▶ *Keeping the front of your foot on the floor, slowly move the ball from side to side in front of the heel.*

▶ *Continue Gliding the ball from side to side as you work your way to the back of the heel and then back to point 5.*

Shear

▶ *With the ball on point 5, use a slightly heavier compression to wiggle your foot left to right. The ball should barely move.*

Rinse

▶ *Place the ball on point 2, directly under the big toe knuckle. Apply tolerable compression to that point, then press the ball toward your heel in a continuous motion with tolerable, consistent pressure.*

▶ *Lift your foot to move to the next knuckle. Repeat from each one.*

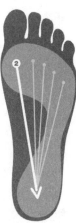

Friction

▶ *Using light, quick, random movements, rub your foot and toes over the ball in a scribble-like motion.*

Body Scan Reassess

▶ *When you finish this self-treatment on one foot, close your eyes and use your Body Sense to quickly notice whether you sense any changes in your leg. Repeat all the techniques on the other foot.*

Final Body Scan Reassess

▶ *Now that you've self-treated both feet, close your eyes and use your Body Sense to feel your feet on the floor. Notice your joints. Do your legs feel more cohesive on both sides now? Do you feel more evenly grounded?*

Mini Soft Ball Hand Treatment

Grip Assess	**Finger Rinse**
Glide	**Friction**
Shear	**Grip Reassess**

Grip Assess

▶ *Place a soft ball in one hand and squeeze it 3–4 times as firmly as you can.*

▶ *Then place the ball in the other hand and notice whether your grip feels equal in strength or if you have a stronger grip in one hand than in the other.*

Glide

▶ *Place the soft ball between your hands at the base of your palms to Glide both hands at once. To Glide on one hand only, place the ball on a table or other flat surface.*

▶ *Glide the ball from point 3 across the base of the palm to point 5 and return to point 3 with consistent pressure.*

▶ *Continue back and forth as you take 3–4 focused breaths.*

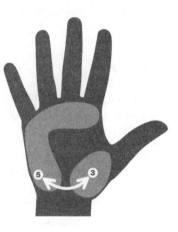

Shear

▶ *Shear by making small circles at the base of your thumb pad, point 3, as you take 3–4 focused breaths. Move slowly and take your time with Shearing, as the thumb pad often carries a lot of stuck stress.*

▶ *Switch hands and repeat.*

Finger Rinse

▶ *Place your left hand flat on the floor or a table. Use the right hand to rub the soft ball over the top of and in between each finger of the left hand in one direction, from the knuckle to the nail. (This also stimulates point 4 on the top hand.)*

▶ *Repeat on the other hand.*

Friction

▶ *Place the ball between your hands and rub lightly in a scribble-like motion. Be sure to include your fingers and wrists.*

Grip Reassess

▶ *Remember what your grip strength felt like when you began, and repeat the Grip Assess by squeezing the soft ball as firmly as you can 3–4 times in each hand. Can you create a more powerful grip with less effort? Does your grip feel more equal from left to right?*

14

MELT as Complementary Self-Care

Whether you have acute or chronic pain caused by an injury or surgery, have been diagnosed with a disorder or disease, or are pregnant or have recently had a baby, you are probably wondering whether MELT can help and if it is safe. The answers are yes and yes.

Regardless of what you are currently experiencing, MELT will help improve your body's healing potential and reduce the accumulated stress that occurs when your body endures any of these circumstances and the related medical treatments. Furthermore, MELT complements all forms of medical, pharmaceutical, and alternative care, yet it is not a replacement for or alternative to these direct interventions.

Because stuck stress accumulates in everyone, every day, imagine what your body has to manage when you add the stress of trauma, disease, or pregnancy. Your Autopilot has to manage incoming demands on top of an internal environment that is under chronic, sometimes extreme duress. Pain—your body's warning sign that it needs help—is inevitable, and symptoms become chronic. Increasing inflammation causes further accumulation of stuck stress in the nervous and connective tissue systems, which exacerbates symptoms and hinders your body's ability to repair itself.

Your body's energy is depleted from constantly trying to deal with the barrage of unavoidable internal and external stressors. This leaves little to no energy for healing when you need it most.

This is where MELT comes in. MELT is going to help you reduce the accumulated stress, inflammation, and resulting energy drain. This creates a rebalancing effect in your immune response and your Autopilot regulation, two things that get so out of whack when connective tissue dehydration becomes chronic. MELT improves your body's efficiency and ability to repair and heal itself so pain and other symptoms can be addressed and often eliminated.

You're already off to a good start. You've been doing the Rebalance Sequence and the Hand and Foot Treatment to support your Autopilot's return to efficiency. How you proceed with the Rehydrate and Release techniques is important so that you can gain positive, lasting changes without causing unnecessary stress on your connective tissue or nervous systems.

To reduce and eliminate symptoms from these chronic conditions, you will MELT more frequently during the week but for shorter periods of time. Initially, ten minutes will be the *maximum* amount of time you MELT during any session, and in some cases less than this—even if it feels good. You can always MELT again later to boost your body's healing and to support positive change. As you continue to MELT, you'll add new sequences and more time to achieve the desired effect. Within a fairly short period of time you will be able to transition into a maintenance phase, when you'll be able to MELT less frequently to sustain the results.

How long will it take for you to notice changes? As a Hands-Off Bodyworker, sensing change and improvement is part of the self-treatment process. The changes to look for first are those that you assess during your MELT sessions. When your body starts responding to your self-treatment, this shows that it is adaptable and that other, longer-lasting changes are right around the corner.

Next, look for improvements in day-to-day Autopilot regulation. One sign to look for is sleep improvement—you fall asleep and stay asleep more easily and wake up feeling more refreshed than you did before. Another sign is that your energy improves, especially in the afternoon. These changes indicate that your body's regulation, stability, and repair systems will be able to begin addressing the underlying cause of your pain and other symptoms.

The specific changes and their timing will depend on the intensity and duration of your circumstances, current state of efficiency, health history, and age. Consider how long you've had chronic pain and other symptoms. Give your body the time and attention it needs to get better. Now, instead of spending so much energy feeling frustrated about your pain and symptoms, I want you to shift your energy and thoughts toward eliminating these issues. Tell your body every day that you are going to help it and that you're not a victim.

Be patient and stick with it, and your body's healing capacity will amaze you. Remember, MELT isn't a cure for anything and can't "fix" you. MELT supports your body's natural healing process so your body can heal itself and get you out of pain.

▶ Use Your Sense

In addition to using your Body Sense to notice positive changes as you MELT, you also need to pay attention to pain. Remember, no part of MELT should ever hurt, so pain is your barometer for when you are moving too fast or applying too much pressure.

You may not realize that you are pressing too hard because chronic pain dulls your Body Sense. If you sense discomfort, it may even seem like a good thing, like you're finally getting at the thing that's been hurting you. It's a very human instinct to want to cause pain to the thing that's been causing you pain, but that's not how MELT works. Remember, MELT gets results by gently stimulating the connective tissue and nervous systems, not by overstressing them or initiating a pain response.

▶ Healing Transitions

In this chapter there are issue-specific, step-by-step self-treatment plans based on what has worked for my clients, students, and instructors. There are a few considerations to be aware of as you begin your healing process.

It's important to follow the guidelines outlined for your particular circumstance so you don't trigger an unwanted immune response. If your body does launch this immune response, it releases an abundance of stored toxins and waste into your connective tissue and bloodstream, but your body can't eliminate it quickly enough. The result is that you can feel exhausted, have more pain and other symptoms, or feel tired and achy like you're coming down with the flu. Although you can usually recover from it fairly quickly, it depletes your energy and internal resources.

You may have heard this referred to as a healing crisis or crash, but I prefer to call it a healing transition. It is a sign that although you are making positive changes, you are going too fast for your body. This is your cue to slow down and be more gentle with your body.

If you experience such symptoms, this is not a sign that MELT isn't good for you. Instead, what I have found over and over again is that it shows that you have been doing too many moves in one session or applying too much compression on the roller.

It may seem counterintuitive, but if you experience a healing transition, MELT can support you in decreasing symptoms, including pain. MELT will support your Autopilot's ability to eliminate the toxins that are flooding your system. Your body is working hard to repair itself, and continuing to MELT will help you transition more quickly. Remember to drink small amounts of water consistently and to rest—your connective tissue system and bloodstream will be able to process and eliminate the toxins more efficiently.

When you first start MELTing, you also need to be aware that you might temporarily experience a greater sense of pain. This is because your mind-body communication and connection has been heightened, which is necessary for healing and health. Better communication also means that your brain can now pick up the pain signals that have been going off nonstop in your body. These unaddressed pain alerts are part of what caused your mind-body disconnect in the first place.

If a pain increase occurs when you start MELTing, shorten your MELT sessions, use gentle pressure, and tell your body that you are giving it the care it needs. Keep MELTing and know that any increase of pain symptoms usually lasts for only a few days. Focus your intention on the fact that you have found a real solution that has worked for thousands of people with circumstances similar to yours. Your hope and commitment can support your body's healing process. Soon your brain and body will experience less pain than you have experienced in a long time.

▶ Your Complementary Self-Treatment Plan

The MELT self-treatment plans for complementary care fall under the following three main categories:

Pain due to trauma, injury, or surgery

Diagnosed systemic conditions, disorders, and diseases

Pregnancy and postpartum

Regardless of which category you identify with, you can do every technique in this book. However, the frequency and amount of time you spend MELTing and the order and pace at which you add the Rehydrate and Release techniques vary by circumstance.

It may seem as if these guidelines are meant to merely direct you with caution. They're not. Instead they are the protocols that I have found most effective in guiding you back to your body's ability to heal itself and get out of pain in the shortest period of time. Follow the plan and give your body the time and attention it needs so you can live a healthier, pain-free life.

Below are the sequences referenced in your self-treatment plan. The page numbers contain the full instructions for each move with accompanying photographs. To see the moves in action, refer to the MELT Method DVD, available at www.meltmethod.com.

Sequence Guide

▶ Pain Due to Trauma, Injury, or Surgery

Goals:

- Boost healing and reduce pain and stiffness

- Increase the amount of time you are able to sit, move, and rest without pain

- Improve joint and spinal integrity and flexibility

- Reduce swelling and inflammation in joints to improve the healing process

- Increase soft tissue, joint, disk, and spinal support

- Improve your overall balance, stability, and body ease

- Decrease unnecessary adhesion and scarring from surgery

- Support your sleep cycle

- Support physical therapy treatments

- Reduce recovery time and get back to being active faster

To achieve these goals in your area of concern, you will MELT the rest of your body first. Although you may want to immediately go after where it hurts, especially if pain has been present for a long time, I need you to wait. Here's why: if you start on the area of concern, you may get some immediate pain relief, but it won't last and it could make matters worse. Without enough fluid, you can irritate the already inflamed or damaged tissue and actually increase pain.

Your self-treatment plan will guide you so you achieve lasting results quickly. Just follow the treatment plan for your area of concern, and you will be on your way to feeling better. There are five self-treatment plans for pain due to trauma, injury, or surgery, divided by spine and non-spine areas of concern. For spinal diseases and disorders, see page 285.

Spine

- Chronic Neck Pain Self-Treatment Plan

- Chronic Low Back Pain Self-Treatment Plan

Non-spine

- Upper Body Pain Self-Treatment Plan

- Lower Body Pain Self-Treatment Plan

- Pelvis or Hip Pain Self-Treatment Plan

Chronic Neck Pain Self-Treatment Plan

This self-treatment plan is for those who have chronic neck pain from trauma or issues related to (but not limited to) herniations, bulging or slipped disks, spinal fusions, discectomies, laminectomies, pinched nerves, vertebral fractures, back spasms, or whiplash. You may also want to use this plan for migraines and chronic headaches. For the best results, MELT at least three times a week, choosing from the maps listed. Remember, it's best to MELT at the end of your day, up to an hour before bedtime. Once you have been in the maintenance phase for one month, you may try the MELT maps in Chapter 13.

Each time you do a sequence using the MELT Soft Roller, you'll start and end with an assessment. Be sure to turn your head from side to side before and after you MELT so you can feel the changes you make.

Week 1

Soft Ball Hand or Foot Treatment
Rebalance Sequence

Week 2

Soft Ball Hand Treatment
Upper Body Compression Sequence
Upper Body Length Sequence

Weeks 3 to 4

Map 1
Soft Ball Foot Treatment
Lower Body Compression Sequence

Rebalance and Upper Body Length Sequence
Low Back Release Sequence

Map 2

Soft Ball Hand Treatment
Upper Body Compression Sequence
Rebalance and Upper Body Length Sequence
Lower Body Length Sequence

Maintenance Maps

Map 1

Mini Soft Ball Hand Treatment
Upper Body Compression Sequence
Rebalance and Upper Body Length Sequence
Neck Release Sequence

Map 2

Mini Soft Ball Hand or Foot Treatment
Upper Body Compression Sequence
Lower Body Length and Low Back Release Sequence
Rebalance and Upper Body Length Sequence

Chronic Low Back Pain Self-Treatment Plan

This self-treatment plan is for people who have chronic low back pain from trauma or issues related to (but not limited to) herniations, bulging or slipped disks, spinal fusions, discectomies, laminectomies, pinched nerves, vertebral fractures, or back spasms.

For the best results, MELT at least three times a week, choosing from the maps listed. Remember, it's best to MELT at the end of your day, up to an hour before bedtime. In the third week, you'll introduce the Lower Body Length Sequence, which calls for you to lift your hips onto the roller. If you find this challenging, you can either use the MELT Soft Half Roller (which is half as high) or place folded towels under your head and upper back to decrease the distance. Once you have been in the mainte-nance phase for one month, you may try the MELT maps in Chapter 13.

This is the same self-treatment plan used in the recent MELT research study. People with nonspecific low back pain achieved significant changes in the low back tissue, reducing pain and stiffness, and increasing flexibility.

Week 1

Mini Soft Ball Foot Treatment
Rebalance Sequence

Week 2

Map 1
Mini Soft Ball Foot Treatment
Upper Body Compression Sequence
Lower Body Compression Sequence

Map 2
Mini Soft Ball Foot Treatment
Upper Body Compression Sequence
Lower Body Compression Sequence
Rebalance Sequence

Week 3

Map 1
Mini Soft Ball Foot Treatment
Lower Body Length Sequence
Low Back Release Sequence

Map 2
Mini Soft Ball Foot Treatment
Upper Body Compression Sequence
Rebalance Sequence
Lower Body Length Sequence
Low Back Release Sequence

Week 4

Map 1
Mini Soft Ball Foot Treatment
Rebalance Sequence
Lower Body Length and Low Back Release Sequence

Map 2
Mini Soft Ball Foot Treatment
Rebalance Sequence
Upper Body Compression Sequence
Lower Body Length and Low Back Release Sequence

Map 3
Mini Soft Ball Foot Treatment
Upper Body Compression Sequence
Rebalance Sequence

Maintenance Maps

Map 1
Soft Ball Foot Treatment
Upper Body Compression Sequence
Lower Body Length and Low Back Release Sequence

Map 2
Mini Soft Ball Hand or Foot Treatment
Lower Body Compression Sequence
Lower Body Length and Low Back Release Sequence

Add the Rebalance Sequence 1–2 times per week with a maintenance map after the foot treatment or on its own. Continue to follow either map from weeks 3 to 4 once a week.

Upper Body Pain Self-Treatment Plan

This self-treatment plan is for people who have experienced upper body trauma or issues related to (but not limited to) broken or bruised ribs; tendonitis; broken collarbone or arm; torn shoulder labrum, rotator cuff, or bicep tendon; frozen shoulder; carpal tunnel syndrome; tennis elbow; lung or heart surgery; or upper body osteoarthritic conditions. (For neck pain, follow the Chronic Neck Pain Self-Treatment Plan, page 272.) For the best results, MELT at least three times a week, choosing from the maps listed. Remember, it's best to MELT at the end of your day, up to an hour before bedtime. Once you have been in the maintenance phase for one month, you may try the MELT maps in Chapter 13.

Week 1

Soft Ball Hand or Foot Treatment
Rebalance Sequence

Week 2

Map 1
Mini Soft Ball Hand or Foot Treatment
Lower Body Compression Sequence
Lower Body Length Sequence
Rebalance Sequence
Neck Release Sequence

Map 2
Rebalance Sequence
Lower Body Compression Sequence
Lower Body Length and Low Back Release Sequence (be mindful of how you use your arms when you perform these techniques, and remember to keep your shoulders relaxed)
Mini Soft Ball Hand or Foot Treatment

Weeks 3 to 4

Map 1
Mini Soft Ball Hand Treatment
Lower Body Compression Sequence
Upper Body Length Sequence (be mindful when you do the Double Arm Reach, and skip this move if you feel any pain)
Neck Release Sequence

Map 2
Mini Soft Ball Hand Treatment
Upper Body Compression Sequence
Upper Body Length
Neck Release Sequence

Maintenance Maps

Map 1
Mini Soft Ball Hand Treatment
Upper Body Compression Sequence
Rebalance and Upper Body Length Sequence
Neck Release Sequence

Map 2
Upper Body Compression Sequence
Lower Body Length and Low Back Release Sequence
Rebalance and Upper Body Length Sequence
Neck Release Sequence

Add the Soft Ball Foot Treatment or Mini Soft Ball Foot Treatment
1–2 times per week with a map or on its own. Continue to
follow either map from weeks 3–4 once a week.

Lower Body Pain Self-Treatment Plan

This self-treatment plan is for people who have experienced lower body trauma or issues related to (but not limited to) a torn Achilles tendon or meniscus, ACL, or other knee ligament; tendonitis; broken leg; strained leg muscles; IT band syndrome; restless leg syndrome; compartment syndrome; knee replacement; or lower body osteoarthritic conditions. (For low back pain, follow the Chronic Low Back Pain Self-Treatment Plan, page 272.) For the best results, MELT at least three times a week, choosing from the maps listed. Remember, it's best to MELT at the end of your day, up to an hour before bedtime. Once you have been in the maintenance phase for one month, you may try the MELT maps in Chapter 13.

Week 1

Soft Ball Hand or Foot Treatment
Rebalance Sequence

Week 2

Soft Ball Hand or Foot Treatment
Rebalance Sequence
Upper Body Compression Sequence
Lower Body Length Sequence

Weeks 3 to 4

Map 1
Mini Soft Ball Foot Treatment
Rebalance Sequence
Upper Body Compression Sequence
Lower Body Length and Low Back Release Sequence

Map 2
Mini Soft Ball Foot Treatment
Lower Body Compression Sequence
Lower Body Length and Low Back Release Sequence
Rebalance Sequence

Maintenance Maps

Map 1
Lower Body Compression Sequence
Lower Body Length and Low Back Release Sequence
Neck Release Sequence

Map 2
Rebalance Sequence
Upper Body Compression Sequence
Lower Body Compression Sequence
Lower Body Length and Low Back Release Sequence

Pelvis or Hip Pain Self-Treatment Plan

This self-treatment plan is for people who have experienced lower body trauma or issues related to (but not limited to) pelvic pain, torn labrum (hip joint), hip replacements or resurfacing, sciatica, SI dysfunction, fractured tailbone, incontinence, hysterectomy, tumor or cyst removal from the pelvic region, or fibroid removal. (For low back pain, follow the Chronic Low Back Pain Self-Treatment Plan, page 272.) For the best results, MELT at least three times a week, choosing from the maps listed. Remember, it's best to MELT at the end of your day, up to an hour before bedtime. Once you have been in the maintenance phase for one month, you may try the MELT maps in Chapter 13.

Week 1

Soft Ball Hand or Foot Treatment
Rebalance Sequence

Week 2

Map 1
Soft Ball Hand or Foot Treatment
Rebalance Sequence
Upper Body Compression Sequence
Lower Body Length Sequence

Map 2
Soft Ball Hand or Foot Treatment
Rebalance Sequence
Lower Body Compression Sequence
Lower Body Length Sequence

Weeks 3 to 4

Map 1
Mini Soft Ball Hand or Foot Treatment
Rebalance Sequence
Upper Body Compression Sequence

Lower Body Compression Sequence
Neck Release Sequence

Map 2
Mini Soft Ball Hand or Foot Treatment
Lower Body Compression Sequence
Upper Body Compression Sequence
Upper Body Length Sequence
Neck Release Sequence

Maintenance Maps

Map 1
Rebalance and Upper Body Length Sequence
Upper Body Compression Sequence
Lower Body Length and Low Back Release Sequence
Neck Release Sequence

Map 2
Mini Soft Ball Foot Treatment
Upper Body Compression Sequence
Lower Body Compression Sequence
Lower Body Length and Low Back Release Sequence

▶ Diagnosed Systemic Conditions, Disorders, or Diseases

These self-treatment plans are for people who have been diagnosed with neurological or immune disorders, cancer, connective tissue disorders and diseases, metabolic conditions, and spinal diseases or disorders.

Goals:

- Support your nervous system

- Reduce the negative effects of medication

- Improve your sleep cycle

- Support your organ function

- Improve waste elimination

- Reduce the frequency of "bad days" or "crashing"

- Improve your balance, so you can sustain your independence

- Walk with greater ease

- Improve your daily energy

- Reduce the overall stiffness of your joints

There are three self-treatment plans for diagnosed systemic conditions, disorders, or diseases:

- Neurological or Immune Disorders and Cancer Self-Treatment Plan

- Connective Tissue Disorders and Related Diseases Self-Treatment Plan

- Spinal Diseases and Disorders Self-Treatment Plan

Neurological or Immune Disorders and Cancer Self-Treatment Plan

This self-treatment plan is for people with cancer, as well as multiple sclerosis (MS), Parkinson's, dystonia, Bell's palsy, lupus, and other neurological or immune disorders.

If you are on chemo, radiation, or any medications, you are at a much higher risk of experiencing a healing transition. If it happens, just know it's not a bad thing. It's your cue that your cells need more time to reboot and your connective tissue needs more time to adapt.

In the case of active cancer, you can certainly still MELT. Simply follow the instructions listed here and do not use compression techniques on areas where the tumors are located or where you are prone to side effects of cancer treatment such as lymphedema or lipomas.

If you have MS or cancer with lesions on the spine, do the Rebalance Sequence, skipping it only if it is uncomfortable. You can place a soft towel over the roller for extra cushion. These techniques are not contraindicated for these issues. You may, however, need to limit these techniques to five minutes. Use a timer to see if you can manage five minutes on the roller.

I recommend limiting your MELT sessions to ten minutes a day, at least an hour prior to bedtime to start. Then, if you have no crash or unwanted reactions, you can add an additional ten minutes of MELT in the morning.

For systemic issues like those you're dealing with, it's best to break up sequences for the first three to four weeks and monitor how your body reacts twenty-four hours afterward. If you feel fine, add sequences but still limit your time MELTing. You might do only fifteen minutes at a time for the first six months.

We're going to start off slowly, so the first maps don't all contain all Four R's. For the best results, MELT at least three times a week, choosing from the maps listed. Once you have been in the maintenance phase for one month, you may try the MELT maps in Chapter 13.

Week 1

Map 1
Soft Ball Hand or Foot Treatment
Map 2
Rebalance Sequence

Week 2

Map 1
Mini Soft Ball Hand Treatment
Rebalance Sequence

Map 2
Mini Soft Ball Foot Treatment
Rebalance Sequence

Week 3

Map 1
Rebalance Sequence
Mini Soft Ball Hand Treatment
Upper Body Length Sequence

Map 2

Soft Ball Hand Treatment or Mini Soft Ball Hand Treatment

Rebalance and Upper Body Length Sequence

Week 4

Map 1

Mini Soft Ball Hand Treatment

Rebalance and Upper Body Length Sequence

Neck Release Sequence

Map 2

Mini Soft Ball Foot Treatment

Rebalance and Upper Body Length Sequence

Back Thigh Shear (as in the Lower Body Compression Sequence)

Low Back Release Sequence

Weeks 5 to 6

If you are feeling well and experiencing no healing transition, you are ready to try adding compression techniques. Your sessions will now increase in duration by five minutes. Now fifteen minutes is your maximum MELTing time.

Map 1

Mini Soft Ball Hand Treatment

Upper Body Compression Sequence

Rebalance and Upper Body Length Sequence

Lower Body Length Sequence

Neck Release Sequence

Map 2

Mini Soft Ball Foot Treatment

Rebalance and Upper Body Length Sequence

Lower Body Compression Sequence

Lower Body Length and Low Back Release Sequence

If you are sensing positive changes, you can continue to work with these two MELT maps. If you are experiencing symptoms from a healing transition, go back to the maps from week 4 for two weeks and then try again. If your body is managing the Lower and Upper Body Compression Sequences with no added symptoms, you can even bring your MELT sessions up to twenty minutes and move on to the maintenance maps.

Maintenance Maps

Map 1

Mini Soft Ball Hand Treatment

Rebalance and Upper Body Length Sequence

Upper Body Compression Sequence

Neck Release Sequence

Lower Body Length and Low Back Release Sequence

Map 2

Mini Soft Ball Foot Treatment

Lower Body Compression Sequence

Lower Body Length and Low Back Release Sequence

Rebalance and Upper Body Length Sequence

Neck Release Sequence

Connective Tissue Disorders and Related Diseases Self-Treatment Plan

More than two hundred disorders impact connective tissue, including rheumatoid arthritis, chronic fatigue, fibromyalgia, Ehlers-Danlos syndrome, Marfan syndrome, scleroderma, lipomas, and Dupuytren's contracture. Related metabolic diseases include diabetes.

We're going to start off slowly, so the first maps don't all contain all Four R's. For the best results, MELT at least three times a week, choosing from the maps listed. Remember, it's best to MELT at the end of your day, up to an hour before bedtime. Once you have been in the maintenance phase for one month, you may try the MELT maps in Chapter 13.

For chronic fatigue or fibromyalgia or any other connective tissue disorder, the problem is widespread connective tissue damage, neurological distress, and pain.

You must not overdo any self-treatment, whether it's MELT or any other technique. If you "crash," even ten minutes is too much just yet. MELT for five minutes once or twice a day for a week and then try a ten-minute session again.

Weeks 1 to 2

Every day, pick one of the three maps below.
No more than ten minutes per day. Only one per day!

Map 1
Mini Soft Ball Foot Treatment

Map 2
Mini Soft Ball Hand Treatment

Map 3
Rebalance Sequence

Week 3

Rebalance Sequence
Mini Soft Ball Hand or Foot Treatment
Upper Body Length Sequence
Now you are ready to combine sequences!

Week 4

Map 1
Mini Soft Ball Hand Treatment
Rebalance and Upper Body Length Sequence
Neck Release Sequence

Map 2
Mini Soft Ball Foot Treatment
Rebalance and Upper Body Length Sequence
Low Back Release Sequence

Weeks 5 to 6

If you are feeling good and experiencing no healing transitions, you are ready to try adding compression techniques every other day. On the off days, do a Soft Ball Foot Treatment. Your sessions will still last only 10–15 minutes.

Map 1

Rebalance and Upper Body Length Sequence

Upper Body Compression Sequence

Neck Release Sequence

Map 2

Rebalance and Upper Body Length Sequence

Lower Body Compression Sequence (do only the first two areas on the inner thigh)

Low Back Release Sequence

Maintenance Maps

Map 1

Mini Soft Ball Hand Treatment

Rebalance and Upper Body Length Sequence

Upper Body Compression Sequence

Lower Body Length Sequence

Neck Release Sequence

Map 2

Mini Soft Ball Foot Treatment

Lower Body Compression Sequence

Lower Body Length and Low Back Release Sequence

Rebalance and Upper Body Length Sequence

Spinal Diseases and Disorders Self-Treatment Plan

Limit your time on the roller to the ten-minute maps for the first four weeks. You may need to limit the duration of the Rebalance Sequence to five minutes over the first two weeks. Use a timer to see if you can manage five minutes on the roller.

If you have a spinal disorder or disease, we recommend starting off with the MELT Soft Half Roller, which offers you a soft flat side for greater support when you're lying the length of the roller. The Soft Half Roller is available at www.meltmethod.com.

Week 1

Soft Ball Hand or Foot Treatment
Rebalance Sequence

Weeks 2 to 3

Map 1
Rebalance Sequence
Soft Ball Foot Treatment or Mini Soft Ball Foot Treatment
Upper Body Length Sequence

Map 2
Soft Ball Hand Treatment or Mini Soft Ball Hand Treatment
Rebalance and Upper Body Length Sequence

Map 3
Soft Ball Foot Treatment
Lower Body Compression Sequence
Rebalance and Upper Body Length Sequence

Maintenance Maps

Map 1
Mini Soft Ball Hand Treatment
Rebalance and Upper Body Length Sequence
Lower Body Length Sequence
Neck Release Sequence

Map 2
Mini Soft Ball Foot Treatment
Rebalance and Upper Body Length Sequence
Lower Body Compression Sequence
Lower Body Length and Low Back Release Sequence

◗ Pregnancy and Postpartum

The changes a woman's body experiences during forty weeks of pregnancy and what my clients call the long fourth trimester, postpartum, come with challenges. The daily structural changes and fluctuation of hormones affects your organs, joints, posture, sleep, digestion, and mental state. MELT will support your body to better navigate these changes, give you energy, and keep you grounded. If you take a little time to MELT, you will give yourself and your baby a lot of support.

Pregnancy Self-Treatment Plan

The self-treatment plan for pregnancy is laid out by trimester. If you're in your first trimester, start at week one and follow the plan throughout your pregnancy. If you're starting MELT in your second trimester, begin at week one and omit Rib Length from the Upper Body Compression Sequence. If you're starting in your third trimester, repeat the options for week one for the remainder of your pregnancy.

Goals:

- Prepare your body for the many changes you will experience in each trimester

- Keep your pelvis supple yet stable through each trimester

- Sustain diaphragmatic movement as your abdominal organs shift upward

- Reduce common symptoms of heartburn, constipation, and acid reflux

- Maintain integrity in your spine

- Reduce hand and foot swelling

- Support your sleep cycle and get a more restful night's sleep

- Support your changing body shape and ease into new structural adaptations that are inevitable during pregnancy

- Sustain a good connection to your shifting center of gravity to reduce neck and low back pain and damage

We're going to start off slowly, so the first maps don't all contain all Four R's. For the best results, MELT at least three times a week, choosing from the maps listed. Remember, it's best to MELT at the end of your day, up to an hour before bedtime. Once you have been in the maintenance phase for one month, you may try the MELT maps in Chapter 13.

First Trimester

Week 1

Soft Ball Hand or Foot Treatment
Rebalance Sequence

Week 2

Map 1
Soft Ball Hand and Foot Treatment

Map 2
Rebalance Sequence
Upper Body Compression Sequence
Upper Body Length Sequence

Map 3
Lower Body Compression Sequence
Lower Body Length Sequence

Week 3 Until the End of Your First Trimester

Map 1
Soft Ball Foot Treatment
Lower Body Compression Sequence
Low Back Release Sequence
Rebalance and Upper Body Length Sequence

Map 2
Rebalance and Upper Body Length Sequence
Upper Body Compression Sequence
Neck Release Sequence
Soft Ball Hand Treatment

Second Trimester

Note that the Rib Length move in the Upper Body Compression Sequence has been removed in the second trimester.

In the second trimester, you may want to work with the MELT Soft Half Roller for the Lower Body Length and Low Back Release Sequence. The Soft Half Roller is available at www.meltmethod.com.

Map 1
Mini Soft Ball Foot Treatment
Upper Body Compression Sequence (no Rib Length Assess or Reassess)
Rebalance and Upper Body Length Sequence
Lower Body Length and Low Back Release Sequence
Neck Release Sequence

Map 2
Soft Ball Foot Treatment
Lower Body Compression Sequence
Lower Body Length and Low Back Release Sequence
Rebalance and Upper Body Length Sequence

Map 3
Rebalance and Upper Body Length Sequence
Upper Body Compression Sequence (no Rib Length Assess or Reassess)
Neck Release Sequence
Soft Ball Hand Treatment

Third Trimester

Try this sequence in your third trimester, as the baby begins to occupy more space and the weight of your body increases. Note that there is no Lower Body Length and Low Back Release Sequence.

Map 1
Mini Soft Ball Foot or Hand Treatment
Lower Body Compression Sequence
Rebalance and Upper Body Length Sequence (Limit your time on the roller if you are uncomfortable lying on the roller in the third trimester. Unlike lying on the floor, this is not unsafe.)
Neck Release Sequence

Map 2
Mini Soft Ball Hand or Foot Treatment
Upper Body Compression Sequence (no Rib Length Assess or Reassess)
Neck Release Sequence

Postpartum Self-Treatment Plan

The days and weeks following delivery are a great time to start (or continue) your MELT journey. Many women have found that MELT helps their body recover more quickly from pregnancy and birth. Because MELT is so gentle, even before your doctor gives you the okay to return to full activity, you can add MELT to your day. You will find that MELT helps you get out of postpartum pain and get your pre-baby body back faster.

If you've been MELTing throughout your pregnancy, you can continue with no restrictions. The Soft Ball Hand and Foot Treatment is a great place to start. Listen to your body to know when you are ready to get on the floor and back on the roller. If you are new to MELT or didn't MELT during your pregnancy, begin with the Getting Started Self-Treatment Plan in Chapter 10.

Goals:

- Help heal soft tissue damage

- Support realignment and restoration of pelvic stability and positioning

- Restore organ placement and good function, including digestive and elimination processes

- Support natural weight loss

- Reduce repetitive neck and shoulder strain from breastfeeding and holding a baby

- Improve the quality of your unavoidably shortened sleep hours

Conclusion

Congratulations! Look how far you've come since you started reading this book. Regardless of why you decided to learn about MELT—to get out of pain; improve your health; or look, feel, or perform better—you've started a new relationship with your body. You've probably already experienced some of the immediate benefits of MELT: less pain, better sleep, more energy, greater ease of movement, increased mental clarity, and a greater sense of well-being. Your body is thanking you for giving it the care it needs.

You've accomplished a lot. You've learned the language and techniques of MELT. You've tried the maps. And now that you know how to MELT, you can fit it into your life with less time and effort. More changes will come just by continuing to MELT for ten minutes, three or more times a week. And you won't have to wonder whether it's working or if you're doing it right. You can see and feel the changes.

When you tell people who haven't tried MELT about your results, they may find it hard to believe that something so simple can make such a difference. You may even surprise yourself with the changes you make. When you feel good, it's easier to be motivated, and change occurs organically. You may find yourself effortlessly making positive choices in other aspects of your life and establishing new, healthy habits. Find and do what works for you.

I've seen people make remarkable changes in their bodies and lives. I've heard the term *life-changing* time and again. You can be one of these success stories just by continuing to care for yourself in this new way. You can change your body and your life.

If you feel MELT has helped you already and you want to tell me, please email me at info@meltmethod.com. I'd love to hear your story and how MELT has made a difference for you.

Although you have come to the end of this book, our journey together is just beginning. I know you are going to have questions, and I have more to share with you. A great place to continue learning is the MELT Method website, www.meltmethod.com. There you will find information, guidance, resources, products, downloadable videos, classes, instructors, training, and a community of Hands-Off Bodyworkers. If you have any questions about MELT, please send an email to info@meltmethod.com. Please also join us on Facebook, as I regularly post information about MELT, news of when I am coming to your area, and helpful tips. The more ways we remain connected, the more success you will have with MELT!

I thank you for learning how to help yourself feel better with MELT, and I look forward to reading your personal success story. Until then, stay healthy, happy, and hydrated—and keep MELTing!

MELT Research Study

The name of the study was "Effect of the MELT Method on the Thoracolumbar Connective Tissue," and the objective was to determine how the thickness and other biomechanical properties of fascial tissue changed in subjects with chronic low back pain as a result of using the MELT Method. The research study was conducted in partnership with the New Jersey Institute of Technology and led by a biomedical engineering grad student, Faria Sanjana, who was advised by the founder of the Fascia Research Society, Tom Findley, Ph.D., and Hans Chaudhry, Ph.D.

The study found that participants who did MELT for four weeks had remarkable results, including reduced pain, increased flexibility, and changes in the connective tissue, including decreased thickening. The control group (who did not MELT) showed no significant changes.

The subjects were men and women 25 to 65 with nonspecific, chronic low back pain:

- 22 subjects for the MELT treatment group

- 22 subjects for the control group

Participants couldn't have a BMI over 30, depression, or an anxiety disorder, and they couldn't have had corticosteroid injections in the spine or a severe low back injury or surgery, among other things.

The methods of testing included using an ultrasound machine, the Oswestry Low

Back Pain Scale, and a forward flexion test, as well as, for the first time, a handheld digital palpation device called a MyotonPRO:

- Ultrasound: used to measure thickness of connective tissue in the low back using testing parameters and analysis previously developed by Helene Langevin, Ph.D.

- MyotonPRO: used to measure biomechanical properties including stiffness, elasticity, tone, and stress relaxation time (recovery time when stress is applied)

Procedure

The research itself took place over four weeks. The research subjects came to the testing facility for two separate sets of measurements, then came back at the end of the study for another set of tests.

- **Initial testing:** Ultrasound, MyotonPRO, flexibility test in hip hinge position, and pain scale

    Followed by:
    MELT group: 30-minute MELT self-treatment while watching a MELT video, and 5 minutes resting prior to retest
    Control group: read or relaxed during same period

- **Immediate retest:** Ultrasound, MyotonPRO, flexibility test in hip hinge position, and pain scale

    Followed by:
    MELT group: 4-week MELT self-treatment protocol
    Control group: no changes to routine

- **Final test:** Initial testing was repeated one month later; MELT group did not MELT on the retest day

Outcomes

We're so excited to report that participants who did MELT for four weeks had remarkable results! You can try the Chronic Low Back Pain Self-Treatment Plan that was used in the study. It starts on page 272.

MELT group:

Significant decrease in pain
-43% immediate   -31% long term

Significant increase in flexibility
+9% immediate   +24% long term

Significant decrease in the thickness of the fascial layers and combined thickness of the subcutaneous and fascial layers
-26% immediate   -34% long term

Significant increase in stress relaxation time in the lower area (below the 12th rib) on the left side of the muscle tissues of the spine
+8% immediate   +7% long term

Decreasing trend in stiffness of muscle tissue of the spine

Control group:

The control group showed no significant changes in pain, flexibility, thickness of the fascial layers, stress relaxation time, or stiffness.
Here's what one of our study participants had to say:

A transformation—at least in my case. Over 20 years I have suffered from back pain and have exhausted every means for relief. Considering back surgery last year and then one day I received a MELT survey study. EVERYTHING has changed. With just 15 minutes each day using hand, feet, and back therapy, each new day I am completely free of back pain—completely free!!! Truly a blessing!!!

–Brad O.

Recommended Reading

Books and Articles

Banes, A. J., M. E. Wall, J. Garvin, and J. Archambault. "Cytomechanics: Signaling to Mechanical Load in Connective Tissue Cells and Role in Tissue Engineering." In *Functional Tissue Engineering,* edited by F. Guilak, D. L. Butler, S. A. Goldstein, and D. J. Mooney, 318–334. New York: Springer-Verlag, 2003.

Biel, Andrew. *Trail Guide to the Body: How to Locate Muscles, Bones, and More.* 3rd ed. Boulder, CO: Books of Discovery, 2005.

Chaitow, Leon. *Soft Tissue Manipulation: A Practitioner's Guide to the Diagnosis and Treatment of Soft Tissue Dysfunction and Reflex Activity.* Rochester, VT: Healing Arts Press, 1988.

Chaitow, L., D. Bradley, and C. Gilbert. *Multidisciplinary Approaches to Breathing Pattern Disorders.* New York: Churchill Livingstone, 2002.

Findley, T., and R. Schleip. *Fascia Research: Basic Science and Implications for Conventional and Complementary Health Care.* Munich: Elsevier, 2007.

Franklin, Eric. *Dynamic Alignment Through Imagery.* Champaign, IL: Human Kinetics, 2012.

Greenman, Philip E. *Principles of Manual Medicine.* 2nd ed. Baltimore, MD: Lippincott, Williams & Wilkins, 1996.

Kapandji, I. A. *The Physiology of the Joints.* New York: Churchill Livingstone, 1971.

Kendall, F. P., E. K. McCreary, and P. G. Provance. *Muscles: Testing and Function.* 4th ed. Baltimore, MD: Lippincott, Williams & Wilkins, 1993.

Lindsay, Mark. *Fascia: Clinical Applications for Health and Human Performance.* Independence, KY: Delmar Cengage Learning, 2008.

Madore, A., and J. R. Kahn. "Therapeutic Massage in Integrative Pain Management." In *Integrative Pain Medicine: The Science and Practice of Complementary and Alternative Medicine in Pain Management,* edited by J. Audette and A. Bailey, 353–378. New York: Humana Press, 2008.

Myers, Thomas W. *Anatomy Trains: Myofascial Meridians for Manual and Movement Therapists.* Edinburgh: Elsevier, 2001, 2009.

Upledger, John E. *Craniosacral Therapy: Touchstone for Natural Healing.* Seattle: Eastland Press, 1999.

Weintraub, William. *Tendon and Ligament Healing: A New Approach Through Manual Therapy.* Berkeley, CA: North Atlantic Books, 1999.

Yoo, H., D. R. Baker, C. M. Pirie, B. Hovakeemian, and G. H. Pollack. "Characteristics of Water Adjacent to Hydrophilic Interfaces." In *Water: The Forgotten Biological Molecule,* edited by D. LeBihan and H. Fukuyama, 123–136. Singapore: Pan Stanford, 2011.

Research Papers and Abstracts

Aukland, K., and R. K. Reed. "Interstitial-Lymphatic Mechanisms in the Control of Extracellular Fluid Volume." *Physiological Reviews* 73, no. 1 (1993): 1–78.

Banes, A., A. J. Banes, J. Qi, J. Dmochowski, D. Bynum, M. Schramme, and M. Patterson. "Tenomodulin Is Down-Regulated in Wounded and Strained Bioartificial Equine Tendons In Vitro." Paper presented at the 57th Annual Meeting of the Orthopaedic Research Society, Long Beach, CA, January 2011.

Borgini, E., A. Stecco, J. A. Day, and C. Stecco. "How Much Time Is Required to Modify a Fascial Fibrosis?" *Journal of Bodywork and Movement Therapies* 14, no. 4 (2010): 318–325.

Bouffard, N. A., K. R. Cutroneo, G. J. Badger, S. L. White, T. R. Buttolph, H. P. Ehrlich, D. Stevens-Tuttle, and H. M. Langevin. "Tissue Stretch Decreases Soluble TGF-Beta1 and Type-1 Procollagen in Mouse Subcutaneous Connective Tissue: Evidence from Ex Vivo and In Vivo Models." *Journal of Cellular Physiology* 214, no. 2 (2008): 389–395.

Bove, G. M. "Focal Nerve Inflammation Induces Neuronal Signs Consistent with Symptoms of Early Complex Regional Pain Syndromes." *Experimental Neurology* 219, no. 1 (2009): 223–227.

Bove, G. M., W. Weissner, and M. F. Barbe. "Long Lasting Recruitment of Immune Cells and Altered Epi-Perineurial Thickness in Focal Nerve Inflammation Induced by Complete Freund's Adjuvant." *Journal of Neuroimmunology* 213 (2009): 26–30.

Chaitow, L. "Chronic Pelvic Pain: Pelvic Floor Problems, Sacroiliac Dysfunction and the Trigger Point Connection." *Journal of Bodywork and Movement Therapies* 11 (2007): 327–339.

Chaudhry, H., Z. Ji, N. Shenoy, and T. Findley. "Viscoelastic Stresses on Anisotropic Annulus Fibrosus of Lumbar Disk under Compression, Rotation, and Flexion in Manual Treatment." *Journal of Bodywork and Movement Therapies* 13, no. 2 (2009): 182–191.

Day, J. A., C. Stecco, and A. Stecco. "Application of Fascial Manipulation Technique in Chronic Shoulder Pain—Anatomical Basis and Clinical Implications." *Journal of Bodywork and Movement Therapies* 13, no. 2 (2009): 128–135.

Dilley, A., and G. M. Bove. "Resolution of Inflammation Induced Axonal Mechanical Sensitivity and Conduction Slowing in C-Fiber Nociceptors." *Journal of Pain* 9, no. 2 (2008): 185–192.

Falla, D., G. Jull, T. Russell, B. Vicenzino, and P. Hodges. "Effect of Neck Exercise on Sitting Posture in Patients with Chronic Neck Pain." *Physical Therapy* 87, no. 4 (2007): 408–417.

Ferreira, M. L., P. H. Ferreira, and P. W. Hodges. "Changes in Postural Activity of the Trunk Muscles Following Spinal Manipulative Therapy." *Manual Therapy* 12, no. 3 (2007): 240–248.

Gabbiani, G. "Evolution and Clinical Implications of the Myofibroblast Concept." *Cardiovascular Research* 38, no. 3 (1998): 545–548.

Holm, S., A. Indahl, and M. Solomonow. "Sensorimotor Control of the Spine." *Journal of Electromyography and Kinesiology* 12, no. 3 (2002): 219–234.

James, H., L. Castaneda, M. E. Miller, and T. Findley. "Rolfing Structural Integration Treatment of Cervical Spine Dysfunction." *Journal of Bodywork and Movement Therapies* 13, no. 3 (2009): 229–238.

Langevin, H. M. "Connective Tissue: A Body-Wide Signaling Network?" *Medical Hypotheses* 66, no. 6 (2006): 1074–1077.

Langevin, H. M., C. J. Cornbrooks, and D. J. Taatjes. "Fibroblasts Form a Body-Wide Cellular Network." *Histochemistry and Cell Biology* 122, no. 1 (2004): 7–15.

Langevin, H. M., J. R. Fox, C. Koptiuch, G. J. Badger, A. C. Greenan-Naumann, N. A. Bouffard, et al. "Reduced Thoracolumbar Fascia Shear Strain in Human Chronic Low Back Pain." *BMC Musculoskeletal Disorders* 12 (2011): 203.

Lee, D. G., L. J. Lee, and L. McLaughlin. "Stability, Continence, and Breathing: The Role of Fascia Following Pregnancy and Delivery." *Journal of Bodywork and Movement Therapies* 12, no. 4 (2008): 333–348.

Lee, D. G., and A. Vleeming. "Impaired Load Transfer Through the Pelvic Girdle—A New Model of Altered Neutral Zone Function." Paper presented at the 3rd Interdisciplinary World Congress on Low Back and Pelvic Pain, Vienna, Austria, 1998.

Leusen, I. "Regulation of Cerebrospinal Fluid Composition with Reference to Breathing." *Physiology Review* 52 (1972): 1–56.

Liebsch, D. "Fascia Is Able to Actively Contract and Thereby to Influence Musculoskeletal Mechanics." Paper presented at the 5th World Congress of Biomechanics, Munich, Germany, July–August 2006.

O'Rourke, C., I. Klyuzhin, J. S. Park, and G. H. Pollack. "Unexpected Water Flow Through Nafion-Tube Punctures." *Physical Review E: Statistical, Nonlinear, and Soft Matter Physics* 83, no. 5 (2011).

Pollack, G. H. "Water, Energy and Life: Fresh Views from the Water's Edge." *International Journal of Design & Nature and Ecodynamics* 5, no. 1 (2010): 27–29.

Qi, J., L. Chi, D. Bynum, and A. J. Banes. "Gap Junctions in IL-1beta-Mediated Cell Survival Response to Strain." *Journal of Applied Physiology* 110, no. 5 (2011): 1425–1431.

Reed, R. K., A. Lidén, and K. Rubin. "Edema and Fluid Dynamics in Connective Tissue Remodelling." *Journal of Molecular and Cellular Cardiology* 48, no. 3 (2010): 518–523.

Schleip, R. "Fascial Plasticity—A New Neurobiological Explanation: Part 1." *Journal of Bodywork and Movement Therapies* 7, no. 1 (2003): 11–19.

———. "Fascial Plasticity—A New Neurobiological Explanation: Part 2." *Journal of Bodywork and Movement Therapies* 7, no. 2 (2003): 104–116.

Schleip, R., W. Klingler, and F. Lehmann-Horn. "Active Fascial Contractility: Fascia May Be Able to Contract in a Smooth Muscle-Like Manner and Thereby Influence Musculoskeletal Dynamics." *Medical Hypotheses* 65, no. 2 (2005): 273–277.

Schleip, R., I. L. Naylor, D. Ursu, W. Melzer, A. Zorn, H. J. Wilke, F. Lehmann-Horn, and W. Klingler. "Passive Muscle Stiffness May Be Influenced by Active Contractility of Intramuscular Connective Tissue." *Medical Hypotheses* 66, no. 1 (2006): 66–71.

Shah, J. P., J. V. Danoff, M. J. Desai, S. Parikh, Y. Nakamura, T. M. Phillips, and L. H. Gerber. "Biochemicals Associated with Pain and Inflammation Are Elevated in Sites Near to and Remote from Active Myofascial Trigger Points." *Archives of Physical Medicine and Rehabilitation* 89, no. 1 (2008): 16–23.

Sikdar, S., R. Ortiz, T. Gebreab, L. H. Gerber, and J. P. Shah. "Understanding the Vascular Environment of Myofascial Trigger Points Using Ultrasonic Imaging and Computational Modeling." Paper presented at the 32nd Annual International Conference of the Institute of Electrical and Electronics Engineers, Engineering in Medicine and Biology Society, Buenos Aires, Argentina, August–September 2010.

Sikdar, S., J. P. Shah, E. Gilliams, T. Gebreab, and L. H. Gerber. "Assessment of Myofascial Trigger Points (Mtrps): A New Application of Ultrasound Imaging and Vibration Sonoelastography." Paper presented at the 32nd Annual International Conference of the Institute of Electrical and Electronics Engineers, Engineering in Medicine and Biology Society, Vancouver, Canada, August 2008.

Stecco, A., V. Macchi, C. Stecco, A. Porzionato, J. Ann Day, V. Delmas, and R. De Caro. "Anatomical Study of Myofascial Continuity in the Anterior Region of the Upper Limb." *Journal of Bodywork and Movement Therapies* 13, no. 1 (2009): 53–62.

Stecco, A., A. Meneghini, R. Stern, C. Stecco, and M. Imamura. "Ultrasonography in Myofascial Neck Pain: Randomized Clinical Trial for Diagnosis and Follow-up." *Surgical and Radiologic Anatomy* 36 (2014): 243–53.

Stecco, C., P. Pavan, P. Pachera, R. De Caro, and A. Natali. "Investigation of the Mechanical Properties of the Human Crural Fascia and Their Possible Clinical Implications." *Surgical and Radiologic Anatomy* 36 (2014): 25–32.

Stecco, C., V. Macchi, A. Porzionato, A. Morra, A. Parenti, A. Stecco, V. Delmas, and R. De Caro. "The Ankle Retinacula: Morphological Evidence of the Proprioceptive Role of the Fascial System." *Cells, Tissues, Organs* 192, no. 3 (2010): 200 –201.

van der Wal, J. "The Architecture of the Connective Tissue in the Musculoskeletal System: An Often Overlooked Functional Parameter as to Proprioception in the Locomotor Apparatus." *International Journal of Therapeutic and Massage Bodywork* 2 (2009): 9–23.

DVDs

Guimberteau, Jean-Claude, MD. *Strolling Under the Skin (Promenade sous la peau): Images of Living Matter Architectures* DVD. Directed by Jean-Claude Guimberteau. Amsterdam: Elsevier, 2004.

Hedley, Gil. *Integral Anatomy Series.* DVD series. Beverly Hills, FL: Integral Anatomy Productions, n.d.

Websites

Anatomy Trains, Thomas Myers, www.anatomytrains.com

Fascia Research, Robert Schleip, www.fasciaresearch.com

J. C. Guimberteau, www.guimberteau-jc-md.com/en

Integral Anatomy, Gil Hedley, www.integralanatomy.com

Diane Lee, www.dianelee.com

Other research papers, abstracts, and posters regarding fascial contractility, responsiveness, hydration, and other compelling concepts and studies can be found at www.fasciaresearch.com and www.fasciacongress.org.

Acknowledgments

I would like to dedicate this book to my mentors, clients, and students, who have been my teachers and allowed me to become one. I have not traveled down this road alone. I have so many people to thank for their unending belief, trust, guidance, and teaching.

Thank you to my writing partner and collaborator in all things MELT, Debbie Karch. The depth of Debbie's skills and background in training and development have been an invaluable asset in bringing this method to everyone. Debbie has helped make it possible for people to learn complex information from me even if they don't have a background in human science. Her years of dedicated work and friendship are why this book exists in a format usable by anyone.

I am also very blessed and utterly grateful for the support of the growing fascial community that has arisen over the past twenty years. This international community with its pioneering "Rolfers turned researchers" includes some of my greatest allies. Although I wasn't a researcher or clinician, the key players in the world of fascia and progressive human science have welcomed me and informed, challenged, and guided my work. Very special thanks to Jean Pierre Barral, D.O.; Leon Chaitow, D.O., N.D.; Thomas Findley, M.D., Ph.D.; Jean Claude Guimberteau, M.D.; Gil Hedley, Ph.D.; Diane Lee; Tom Myers; and Robert Schleip, Ph.D. I feel privileged to learn this information as you are making the discoveries—long before it will ever be taught in school. Your kindness to me and your contribution to my work can never be repaid.

This community has taken a huge leap because of the vision and drive of Thomas Findley, who has gathered fascial scientists and clinicians from around the world to share the latest and best research on human fascia. His contributions to the MELT research study on chronic low back pain were invaluable.

A very special thank-you to renegade "somanaut" Gil Hedley. As I have seen you blaze your own path in pursuit of what connects us beneath the surface, I have been inspired to make my own path. Your belief in me has propelled me and my work in profound ways. The gratitude I have for you and our friendship is without measure.

Thanks to the dozens of researchers and scientists who have dedicated their lives to expanding the boundaries of traditional research, including Carla and Antonio Stecco, Helene Langevin, Candace Perth, James Oschman, and Gerald Pollack. You have each helped me enrich my education through your books, papers, journals, and articles and have given me tangible evidence to validate what I have observed for more than fifteen years.

I also want to thank each person who allowed me to share my hands-on and hands-off techniques. I have great love and respect for you. Your trust and belief in me is part of the strong foundation MELT is built upon. You teach and inspire me every day.

Thank you to the hundreds of MELT instructors who have spent their time learning and practicing my work with open hearts and minds. You have all been a blessing to me and the hundreds of thousands of people you have helped. I am so grateful, proud, and humbled by your support and love of this method.

A special thanks to Sara Bethell, who has been an invaluable asset as a wise second set of eyes for this book. Debbie and I are grateful for your perfect package of wordsmith and MELT instructor.

Deep gratitude to the rest of my team for your help in building the foundation of the MELT universe. Your talents and support of the business have made it possible for me to do what I love and for MELT to reach a wider audience.

This book would not exist if it weren't for Mark Tauber, senior vice president and publisher, and the entire team at HarperOne, as well as Heidi Krupp-Lisiten, owner of Krupp Kommunications. Thank you for sharing my vision that MELT can be a force in changing how people care for themselves and live a pain-free life.

Thank you to Phil Widlanski. I am forever grateful for your generosity, and my office door is always open to you.

I would not be where I am without my lifelong friends Brian Leighton and Darren Lisiten, who somehow are always there to advise me so I don't have to "learn things the hard way." Their unconditional support keeps me on solid ground and reminds me that the path my life travels is the right one.

I am so appreciative for the support of my husband, mom, family, and closest friends who have always unconditionally encouraged my passion and pursuits. I am a better person because of your belief and love.

Index

headaches, 13, 28, 38, 43, 50, 51, 119–121, 130; self-care plan, 271–272

healing crisis/transitions, 267–268

health benefits of MELT, 37–38, 42–44, 50–51, 53–54, 150, 225–226

heart surgery, 275; self-care plan, 275–276

Hedley, Gil, ix–xi, 4, 23, 24, 26, 99

herniations, 80, 271, 272; self-care plan, 271–272, 272–274

hip: replacements or resurfacing, 278; self-care plan, 278–279; torn labrum, 278

hip pain self-treatment plan, 278–279

Hip to Heel Press, 114–115, 190–191, 250–251

human dissection, 4, 23–24, 25, 99

hydration, 16, 26–27, 30, 32, 34–35, 42–44. *See also* Rehydrate; water

hysterectomy, 278; self-care plan, 278–279

ideal alignment, 60–61, 64, 65–66

imbalance: ideal alignment vs. common imbalances, 65–67; misunderstanding of muscle, 20–21. *See also* misalignment; NeuroCore system; Rebalance; regulation

immune disorders, 279; self-care plan, 279–283

incontinence, 278; self-care plan, 278–279

indirect Shearing, 101, 104, 108

inflammation, 33–34, 44, 50; compression and joint, 33–34, 122–123. *See also* compression; connective tissue; connective tissue dehydration; regulation

Inner and Back Thigh Rinse, 184, 245

Inner Thigh Glide and Shear, 180–182, 243–244

IT band, 96, 276; self-care plan, 276–277

joints: damage to, 33–34, 122–123; Hand and Foot Treatment of, 130–133, 134–136; misalignment and compression of, 20–21, 27, 29–30, 33–34, 50; stabilization of, 31–32

knee ligament, 276; self-care plan, 276–277

knee pain, 96, 121, 123, 132, 143, 173; self-care plan, 276–277

knee replacement, 276; self-care plan, 276–277

laminectomies, 271, 272; self-care plan, 271–272, 272–274

Langevin, Helene, 294

leg: broken, 276; self-care plan, 276–277; strained muscles, 276

length techniques. *See* Two-Directional Length techniques

lipomas, 280, 283; self-care plan, 283–285

Low Back Decompress, 220–221, 252

low back pain, 43, 120, 122, 135, 143, 211, 270, 272, 287; self-care plan, 272–274

Low Back Release Sequence, 217–221

Lower Body Compression Sequence, 174–185, 241–246

Lower Body Length and Low Back Release Sequence, 248–252

Lower Body Length Sequence, 186–191

Lower Body Pain Self-Treatment Plan, 276–277

lung surgery, 275; self-care plan, 275–276

lupus, 280; self-care plan, 280–283

lymph drainage therapy, 52

lymphedema, 280

manual therapy: MELT inspiration, 27, 35, 52, 98–102, 104, 130; practice, 4, 11; Rolfing, 25–26, 96

Marfan syndrome, 283; self-care plan, 283–285

massage, 97

"masses" of the body, 61, 64–66; Autopilot and, 76; length techniques and, 113, 117; origin of, 60–62; tip for compressing, 112

medical treatment: cures, 18–19; limitations for pain, 14, 18–20, 34, 43–44; using MELT with, 265, 279–280

MELT maps, 54, 68, 147, 225–228; Fifteen- to Twenty-Minute Maps, 230; Ten-Minute Maps, 229. *See also* sequence guide

meniscus, torn, 276; self-care plan, 276–277

metabolic disorders, 279; self-care plan, 279–280

migraines, 18, 130, 271; self-care plan, 271–272

Mini Soft Ball Foot Treatment, 140–143, 260–261

Mini Soft Ball Hand Treatment, 137–139, 262–263

misalignment, 20–21, 29–30, 33, 64, 80, 123. *See also* alignment; ideal alignment; imbalance

movement: connective tissue system role in, 30–32; differentiation of, 79, 117; how adequate hydration improves, 32. *See also* repetitive movements/postures

moves, 54, 72, 148, 231

multiple sclerosis, 280; self-care plan, 280–283

muscles: brain communication with, 30–31, 32; connective tissue and, 20–21, 29–30; how dehydration negatively affects, 30; imbalance and, 20–21, 80; stability and, 78–79

Myers, Tom, 26, 133